yellow light moments

MAXIMIZE YOUR HEALTH AND VITALITY THROUGH THE POWER OF PAUSING

Jennie Phillips, MSEd

broad book press

Broad Book Press, Publisher
Cover and interior design by Andrew Welyczko, AbandonedWest Creative, Inc.
Author photography by Kayla Colwell McGee

Copyright © 2024 by Jennie Phillips

All rights reserved.
No part of this publication may be reproduced, distributed, or transmitted in any form or by any means, including photocopying, recording, or other electronic or mechanical methods, without the prior written permission of the publisher, except in the case of brief quotations embodied in critical reviews and certain other noncommercial uses permitted by law. For permission requests, write to the publisher, subject line "Attention: Permissions" at info@broadbookgroup.com

Paperback ISBN: 978-1-963-549-16-4
eBook ISBN: 978-1-963-549-17-1

Published in the United States by Broad Book Press, an imprint of Broad Book Group, Edwardsville, IL.

Library of Congress Control Number: 2024917313

This book is dedicated to:

Julia, Brian, and Jessica,

My amazing children. Words cannot fully capture the depth of my feelings for each of you. I am ridiculously proud of who you are and who you are becoming. You fill my life with joy, wonder, and purpose. You are my greatest adventure, my reason for pushing forward, my source of hope in challenging times, and the loves of my life. You are my strength and my inspiration. Each moment with you is a gift and I thank God for you every day.

Thank you for being the incredible individuals you are and for making my life so rich and meaningful. I love you more than words can say!

With all my heart,

Mom

Dr. Bob Buckman,

My unwavering support, my mentor, my friend. You went beyond medical diagnoses and treatment and poured yourself into me addressing my heart, head, and body. Thank you for your wisdom, love, and friendship. I am deeply grateful for your endless support and encouragement throughout my journey. Your belief in me has been a constant source of strength, lifting me up when I needed it most and guiding me through every challenge and triumph.

Thank you for being an irreplaceable part of my life. I cherish every moment together, especially those spent sharing blueberry pancakes.

With all my love and gratitude,

XOXO

TESTIMONIALS

Jennie Phillips' *Yellow Light Moments* is a profound exploration of life's pivotal pauses—the moments that compel us to slow down, reflect, and recalibrate. As a certified fitness professional holding a Master of Education degree, Jennie provides invaluable insights, offering readers practical tools and strategies to learn from these moments and grow stronger, both personally and professionally. Through expert guidance, Jennie empowers clients and readers alike to embrace challenges, find clarity, and turn obstacles into opportunities for growth. Her compassionate and relatable approach makes this book a must-read for anyone seeking to navigate life's transitions with intention and grace.

SARA KOOPERMAN, JD and CEO of SCW Fitness Education

As a 50-year-old father of four active young adults currently in high school and college, life can be chaotic. And with a full-time professional career, a retail brick-and-mortar small business owner, and opening of the largest restaurant and pub in my city, I have more candles burning at more ends than I can currently keep track of. Any fractions of time remaining in my schedule are hardly ever used to invest in myself through self-care, nutrition management, or strength training and exercise which led to a 30-year decline from competitive athlete all the way down to sluggish, lifeless, middle-aged, dad-bod fat guy. That was until Jennie came into my life and changed it all. *Yellow Light Moments* is a testimony to the life that Jennie lives, and the life she inspired in ME! Not only have I lost nearly 40 pounds but the lessons in this book surrounding goal planning, accountability, action plans, and filtering out all the distractions in life that constantly compete for your attention, were the solutions I was seeking for so long. I transformed my body, my personal relationships improved, I have a stronger presence in my family life, and even my career has flourished by implementing her strategies. It's cliché, but body AND soul were impacted.

ADAM MICUN, Health and Safety Executive, Entrepreneur, Restaurateur, Father of Four

As a business owner and mom of four, I find *Yellow Light Moments* to be an invaluable resource that I can reference frequently. The book simplifies and organizes crucial life priorities that are often overshadowed by an overbooked schedule. Its exercises provide an honest assessment of both physical and mental health, revealing how our daily choices impact productivity and overall well-being. Jennie offers clear guidance on managing day-to-day decisions to achieve a healthier life.

MICHELLE MOTLEY, Mom of Four and Owner of Source Juicery

Through personal experiences and the backing of scientific studies, Phillips provides an explanation on why we often need to take the time to reflect on our lives and what is going well and what could be improved. This book provides all the tools necessary to make authentic changes for the better. If you're looking for something to help guide you through some life changing decisions, *Yellow Light Moments* is the perfect resource.

PAUL VANDERSTEEN, Retired Science Teacher and Science Department Chair, Owner of Coach Steen Running

I've been here, the moment of confusion, exhaustion, and self disappointment; but I never knew what these moments were trying to tell me. I hadn't thought through what my mind, body and soul were trying to teach me. *Yellow Light Moments* has brightened up my mind to all the hints I've missed or even ignored. This book provides the reminders of how a fast-paced life effects us, and how the important part, our health and wellness, plays into that. This book helps guide us to *evaluate, empower, engage, execute and enjoy* the life and lifestyle we want.

JENNIFER HOPPES, Elementary Educator

Jennie is not retelling something she learned in a class or a seminar. She is sharing the process she undertook to amplify the joy, balance, and vitality in her life. And what she discovered was pretty amazing. There is no right answer for everyone, but by asking yourself the right questions, and taking the time to prioritize what is important, you can develop your personal formula to increase the joy, balance and vitality in your life.

SCOTT TOMER, Entrepreneur and Business Coach

I have never seen a book that breaks lifestyle improvements down into easy-to-digest facts, the reasons why, and what can be done with your habits to gain better overall health nearly as well as this book. If you want to take control, or take greater control over your life, this is the book for you. It is much more than a self-help book. It is a guide to understanding the fundamental needs your body has, how to understand them and take action, with guided steps and practical ideas along the way. It is a way to be proactive and live your life by design.

ROB RUBBELKE, Wealth Management Advisor

Yellow Light Moments by Jennie Phillips is more than just a guide; it is a powerful catalyst for change and an invaluable addition to the library of anyone seeking to enhance their well-being and productivity. It offers profound insights and practical strategies that are essential for sustaining long-term success and personal fulfillment. As an executive coach dedicated to fostering professional excellence and personal growth, I wholeheartedly recommend this book to anyone committed to achieving their highest potential.

MEGAN MARTIN, Executive Coach and Business Consultant

CONTENTS

Disclaimer xi
Introduction: The Power Of A Yellow Light Moment 1

PART I   **EVALUATE** 13
Chapter 1   The Vitality Evaluation............................ 15
               The Vitality Self-Evaluation 18
Chapter 2   Are You Stable? 23

PART II   **EDUCATE** 27
Chapter 3   Find Your Zzzs 29
Chapter 4   Focus On Your Fork 47
Chapter 5   Self-Care Is A Necessity 85
Chapter 6   Movement Is Key 105

PART III   **EMPOWER** 129
Chapter 7   The Power Of Commitment 131
               My Commitment Page 146
Chapter 8   It Is You Against You 147

PART IV   **ENGAGE** 165
Chapter 9   Proximity Is Power 167

PART V   **ENDING** 171
Chapter 10   My Final Thoughts 173
Epilogue   A New Motto 177

About The Author 179

PART VI   EXECUTE (YOUR YELLOW LIGHT MOMENT WORKBOOK)......................181

Worksheet A	Your Golden Nuggets............................182
Worksheet B	The Vitality Self-Evaluation....................186
Worksheet C	Yellow Light Moment to Find Your Zzzs 193
Worksheet D	Food Diary.......................................194
Worksheet E	Meal Planners 197
Worksheet F	Grocery List Organizer 200
Worksheet G	Grocery Shopping Checklist 201
Worksheet H	Yellow Light Moment to Focus on Your Fork 203
Worksheet I	Time Chunking Your Day........................204
Worksheet J	Yellow Light Moment Journal Page..............205
Worksheet K	Blank Journal Page 206
Worksheet L	Writing Your Mantra 207
Worksheet M	Saying "No" 208
Worksheet N	28 Days to Declutter Your Home Checklist 211
Worksheet O	Yellow Light Moment to Self-Care Is A Necessity...213
Worksheet P	Movement Questionnaire 214
Worksheet Q	Record Your Waist-to-Hip Ratio 215
Worksheet R	Record Your 30 Second Sit-to-Stand Test 216
Worksheet S	Yellow Light Moment to Movement Is Key 217
Worksheet T	Set Your Goals 218
Worksheet U	Mind Map Your Challenges.....................219
Worksheet V	Who You Want to Be............................221
Worksheet W	Discover Your Why 222
Worksheet X	Measure So You Can Manage 223
Worksheet Y	Control Your Controllables......................224
Worksheet Z	Do The Dailies 228
Worksheet AA	Prepare Your If...Then Statements 229
Worksheet BB	Declare Your Non-Negotiables 230
Worksheet CC	Habit Stacking..................................231
Worksheet DD	Habit Tracker 232
Worksheet EE	Identify Your Associations and Collaborations ...233
Worksheet FF	The Vitality Scorecard..........................234
Worksheet GG	Three-Month Refresher........................236

DISCLAIMER

THE CONTENT IN THIS BOOK is intended for educational and informational purposes only and should not be considered a substitute for professional medical advice, evaluation, diagnosis, or treatment. Always seek the advice of your physician, licensed therapist, specialist, or registered dietitian before starting any new treatment or discontinuing an existing treatment.

Sleep
The tips and recommendations for improving sleep hygiene are intended to promote healthy sleep habits and overall well-being. However, individual sleep needs and conditions vary, and chronic sleep issues may require medical evaluation and treatment. If you are experiencing persistent sleep disturbances, insomnia, or any sleep-related disorder, you should consult with a qualified healthcare professional to identify and address underlying causes.

Nutrition
The nutritional information and dietary recommendations offered in this book are general in nature and may not be suitable for everyone. Individual nutritional requirements vary based on factors such as age, gender, health status, and personal preferences. You should seek personalized guidance from a registered dietitian for tailored advice, especially if you have specific dietary needs, allergies, or medical conditions.

Self-Care
The self-care practices discussed in this book are intended to promote holistic well-being and stress management. They are not a replacement

for professional treatment, including mental health treatment or therapy. If you are dealing with severe stress, anxiety, depression, or any mental health condition, it is important to seek assistance from a licensed therapist or mental health professional.

If you or someone you know is struggling or in crisis, help is available. Call or text 988 (The Suicide & Crisis Lifeline) or chat 988lifeline.org.

Exercise

The exercise routines and recommendations in this book are general in nature and may not be suitable for everyone. Prior to starting any new exercise program or making significant changes to your current fitness routine, you should consult with a qualified healthcare provider or fitness trainer, especially if you have any underlying health concerns or medical conditions. It is crucial to consider your individual fitness level, health status, and any pre-existing conditions or injuries before engaging in physical activity. Always listen to your body and modify exercises as needed. Stop any exercise that causes discomfort or pain and seek guidance from a medical provider or qualified fitness professional.

By using this book, you acknowledge and agree that you are responsible for your own health and well-being. The author is not liable for any injury, loss, or damage to you, allegedly arising from any information or suggestions presented here. This book is not intended to be used, nor should it be used, to diagnose or treat any medical or psychological condition. You are solely responsible for your own healthcare decisions and should use your discretion when implementing any practices discussed in this book. Always prioritize your health and safety and consult with appropriate professionals for personalized evaluation, diagnosis, treatment, and guidance.

INTRODUCTION

The Power Of A Yellow Light Moment

WE HAVE ALL had those moments in life that can best be described as "hitting a wall." When that happens, you may feel:

- exhausted
- stressed
- sluggish
- anxious
- overwhelmed
- unmotivated
- pressured
- unproductive
- achy

- stiff
- drained
- done
- confused
- uncertain
- nauseous
- unfocused
- disinterested
- unstable

Whether you experience just one or all of these characteristics of "hitting the wall," the fact is few of us are immune to system overload and eventual exhaustion. When you hit that wall, you may not feel like yourself and the idea of progressing forward may seem overwhelmingly difficult. Everyone hits their "wall" at various times in their life and for different reasons. We all have our own breaking point. Ironically, what you could have managed gracefully on one day, might just put you over the edge on a different day. Sometimes those days turn into weeks, and those weeks turn into months of barely hanging on as you are bombarded with increasing options, opportunities, and obligations leading to overloading your system and ending with a breakdown of pure exhaustion. The amount of stress you experience hustling and grinding to achieve your goals while feeling mentally, emotionally, and physically stable and fulfilled can fluctuate during your lifetime. It is not the same from person to person. What is overwhelming for one person, another can handle with confidence. It is important to not dismiss, diminish, or bury these feelings because you are afraid someone might judge the trials in your life as not being "hard enough."

I remember feeling this way and saying to myself, "I live a blessed life, my house did not just get washed away in a hurricane or burn down in a fire, there is no war in my town, I did not grow up experiencing abandonment or abuse as a child, my children are not fighting a terminal illness, I have money to pay the bills. What do I truly have to complain about compared to others who have it worse?" Know that you do not have to experience a natural disaster, a terrific accident, grave trauma, a catastrophic incident, or a horrific life-threatening medical condition to hit a wall. These are not the conditions or events I am referring to in this book. I am referring to the day-to-day stress that might come from a growing to-do list, pressure to meet work deadlines, tackling household responsibilities, navigating family dynamics, balancing schedules, unexpected financial concerns, and/or managing chronic conditions. When life starts to whisper to you "slow down," and ends up screaming at you "pivot your pace!" Suddenly you feel like you cannot keep your head above water. Stress has a way of creeping up on you when events and tasks start to snowball, then boom... you hit that awful wall. Hitting your wall or your limit of mental, emotional, or physical endurance is not giving up, it is not a weakness, it does not need to be compared and justified to others, and it is not failure. It just means you need to pause, rest, and evaluate what internal and/or external factors led to your fatigue. *There is power in pausing.* It can be significant. It can bring meaningful change. It can enlighten you. It can energize you. It can recalibrate you. It can become your catalyst for growth. That pause is what can save you from the wall. It is okay to give yourself permission, and time, to pause in a world full of noise and chaos.

MY OWN YELLOW LIGHT DAY

My personal physician, Dr. Bob Buckman, who is also one of my most influential mentors, once said he could describe me in two words "Oy, vey!" He has said to me on more than one occasion, "I need you to slow down and stop burning the candle at both ends. It is not healthy to keep up the pace you are going and one day your body will tell you that." Sound like something you have heard before? I remember hitting my wall. I was burned out. I felt overloaded. It was a flood of emotions that hit all at one time. I continued to tell myself that I was unlike other people. That I could manage more, do more, push more, take on more, sleep less, and still find the energy and balance to succeed—until one day I couldn't. It was on that day that I broke. After regaining my composure and control, I sat in silence and prayed, "God, it's me and you... I need your help... how do I find a healthy balance between my professional and my personal life? How do I create a new normal in my life where I am not just surviving day to day, but I am thriving in all areas? What needs to change? Where do I start? Because I cannot continue like this." That day became what I would lovingly refer to as my "Yellow Light Day."

I hit my **first** wall on a Monday morning while sitting on a beach. Yes, a beach. Remember, I said it can hit you anywhere, at any time, if the perfect storm is right. Where most people find peace and serenity enjoying the warmth of the sun on their skin, listening to the waves rhythmically roll in and drift out, I found myself uncomfortable with the stillness. I was anxious, overwhelmed, exhausted, and physically nauseous. Here I was sitting in the soft white sand, smelling the salty ocean breeze, watching the seagulls play. It was a sunny eighty-degree February day and my hometown in Illinois, approximately 745 miles away, was experiencing snow and ice. I had just completed a half marathon the day before along the beautiful blue ocean with my girlfriends in Seaside, Florida. This was my fourth day away from work, home, and family. Earlier that morning my girlfriends packed up the van and started their twelve-hour drive back to our snowy state, while I stayed behind two more days before catching a flight out of Destin,

FL, to Washington, DC. I was attending a professional conference later that week for gym owners, personal trainers, and nutritionists. It made more sense to stay in Florida until Wednesday and fly straight from Florida to DC than to drive 12 hours back to Illinois, sleep one night at home, and then fly back out the next morning to DC. By the time I returned home from the conference in DC, I would have been gone a total of ten days and at the time of booking this trip, an extra 48 hours on a beach sounded like a great idea.

 I was surprised when I hit the wall. I truly was not expecting or prepared for the wave of feelings and the sinking sensation that stopped me in my tracks. Four years before this trip, I had flown eighteen hours and 8,782 miles by myself to visit my best friend in Australia. I was gone for two weeks, and there was no wall. What broke me this time? What was the difference? Looking back... my life, my responsibilities, my health, my work hours, my stress level, my push, my sleep, my food, my energy levels, my exercise, my mental health... everything was different. My physical location did not matter. This would have happened anywhere, because it had been building inside of me for quite some time. I had created the perfect storm because I failed to pause. I ignored the whisper. I kept burning the candle at both ends. I was overextending myself by owning and running my gym, working, and training on a crazy schedule. I saw clients fourteen hours a day, caught a quick nap in my office if I had a cancellation, and ate meals on the gym floor in between clients. I did not know how to balance my work life with my personal life. My husband had experienced a career-ending injury which changed our household in a multitude of ways. Our four **amazing** children who bless and enrich my life and joy beyond anything I could write in this sentence, also bring the inevitable stresses, uncertainties, and demands that come with parenting teenagers through this transformative phase of their lives. I was also fighting a progressive autoimmune disease. Every day I pushed myself to ensure the business did not fail, our doors did not close (a valid post-covid fear), my clients felt like they had the most energetic personal trainer and cheerleader imaginable, and my family felt secure, supported, and loved. I made sure the bills were paid both at work and at home, I ran the weekly miles I felt was expected of me as a successful trainer and coach, and ensured my house was clean and organized. However, on the health front, my doctors were **not** happy with the progress of my lupus.

My body's resources were depleted because the pace I set for myself in the daily hustle and grind was not sustainable for me in the long run. I had no margins. At the same time, I didn't know how to proceed differently because of the pressures of life I was feeling. I did not know how to sit on a beach quietly by myself and be at peace. I did not know how NOT to burn the candle at both ends. Sitting still, relaxing alone, with no work, no calls, no schedule, no texts, no commute, no lists, no expectations, no programming, no chores, no parenting, no grocery shopping, no cleaning, no bill paying, no emails was not something I could do. For many people, this would be heaven, but for me, this was anything but normal and very uncomfortable. This was the first time I had ever been alone without responsibilities, to-dos, the push—and all I could think of were my responsibilities, my to-dos, the push, and the people who I love that were not with me—because I did not feel I had the luxury to press the pause button. I was afraid life would start crashing. It was then it hit me and hit me hard—I did not know how to slow down, and something had to change. That is when I took my first **Yellow Light Moment**.

Traditionally, a yellow light is a sign meaning pause, proceed with caution, slow down, decide, check your surroundings, and tap the brakes. That day became a gut check, a movement check, a mind and sanity check, a rest check, a balance check, a faith check, and a life-gauge check. It was on that day I wrote in my journal that I needed to "Marie Kondo my life." Now, for those of you who do not know who Marie Kondo is, she is a Japanese organizing consultant and author. She is famous for her method of collecting everything you have in a specific category, in one space, and then only keeping the items that "spark joy" in your life, decluttering and eliminating the others. I knew I needed to reflect on everything I had going on in my life and decide what sparked joy. If it did not spark joy or add to the balance in my life, then I needed to let it go. It was time for changes and some drastic ones at that. I started by looking at four areas that I knew would make a difference in my life: my sleep, nutrition, self-care, and movement. These were areas I regularly taught my clients to evaluate, yet I was failing to follow my own advice. Since that day on the beach, I expanded this **evaluation** and wrote this book in hopes of helping you "Marie Kondo **your** life."

MY SECOND YELLOW LIGHT MOMENT

As mentally and emotionally draining as my beach day was, it did kick off my Yellow Light Moment and force me to evaluate what was misaligned in my life and identify areas that needed to change to create balance. It was not until I hit my **second** wall that I really started to incorporate all of the changes. Some of us are slow learners. You see, six months after my Yellow Light Moment on the beach I found myself in the emergency room suffering from severe chest pains, the inability to swallow or lay flat in a bed, and a slew of digestive problems. I had officially hit my physical wall. After many doctors and lots of tests, it came down to the same answer that I found on the beach: I still was not balanced and now it was presenting in my physical health, beyond the progress of my lupus. I had identified what changes needed to be made but had not implemented them effectively and completely. You see, *nothing changes if nothing changes.* Now my body was screaming. Looking back, I knew it was my ego that kept me burning my candle at both ends. I honestly believed as a mom and entrepreneur that I was the only one that could do **all the things** that needed to be done to keep our lives and the business running successfully. I kept saying "I'm fine, everything is fine." I felt I had no other choice than to dig deep and push through to continue to perform and please everyone. Hitting my walls gave me the opportunity (well, it actually forced me) to become introspective and ask myself:

- What is my **why** in doing all of this?
- What do I really want?
- Who do I want to be?
- How do I want to feel?
- Why is it important to make these changes?
- What am I willing to say "no" to?
- What brings me joy?
- What really matters?
- How do I maximize my health and vitality?
- What am I going to do differently **this** time, so I do not end up here again?

It was time I started asking myself better questions. It was time I shifted my perspective. This time I wrote on a note card, "I am making a dynamic contract with myself to elevate how I think and how I act in order to balance my family and my work by prioritizing taking care of myself." I specifically wrote "dynamic" because I knew this promise to myself would be a work in progress with constant changes as my life, both personally and professionally, evolved. I took the time to create systems with firmer boundaries and clearer priorities to create my ideal lifestyle so I would feel restored and rejuvenated. I worked on having more compassion and being comfortable with saying "no," even if I felt I was disappointing someone. I began to let go of my need to please others and I started to own my daily practices. Building a foundation for vitality living is not a one-time choice—it is a dynamically changing process. Through this transformation of creating more vitality in your life, you gain strength, energy, vigor, and liveliness in your overall health and wellness, including your physical health, mental well-being, and emotional strength. It is a lifetime journey based on awareness and clarity of everyday choices that create the patterns of your thoughts, feelings, and behaviors. **My goal is to help you be curious, intuitive and mindful regarding your decisions and actions to meet your goals by getting in the habit of asking yourself this *one* question: "Does this choice support the lifestyle I am creating?" This is the Vitality Mindset—to live less out of habit and more out of intent.**

WHAT TO EXPECT IN THIS BOOK

This book became my Yellow Light Moment, and now I hope it becomes yours. It is meant to be **your** gut check, **your** time to tap the brakes, **your** pause, and **your** evaluation to help you find joy, balance, and vitality in your life. This is not intended to diagnose any medical conditions or replace the assessment or treatment by a doctor, dietitian, or licensed therapist. My goal is not to dive into the depths of any one of these topics or to overwhelm you with statistics, research, or article analysis, but instead to provide you with a health and wellness "aha" moment in your journey. The goal is not to lean on perfection but to integrate the lessons of this book to become more aware of yourself and how you can find a better balance in your life.

There are two ways to simplify life:

1. Decide what is important.
2. Let go of what is not.

Let that sink in for a minute because this is a **big** lesson. We are going to accomplish this together as we navigate through the journey of this book. This book will help you:

EVALUATE where you are currently to provide clarity. Completing a Vitality Evaluation is essential for identifying where to pivot and start your new journey. When you perform an evaluation, particularly of your health and wellness, you are gaining insights by assessing the effectiveness and efficiency of what you are currently doing. For the context of this book, your Vitality Evaluation will assess four areas of your health and wellness: sleep, nutrition, self-care, and movement, by asking:

- What is the quality of your (sleep, nutrition, self-care, movement)?
- How important is your (sleep, nutrition, self-care, movement) to you?
- How much time do you spend on (sleep, nutrition, self-care, movement)?
- Do you value your (sleep, nutrition, self-care, movement)?

Taking time to self-analyze these four areas is the power of the Yellow Light Moment. This will be the first pause I am asking you to take to provide transparency on the areas that will make the biggest impact in your life.

EDUCATE yourself with new information and tools for creating balance in your daily practice. Nothing will change your life faster than learning and building new skills or improving on your existing ones. When we learn, we maximize our potential for success by applying content in an engaging and meaningful way. I want to challenge you to read this book with a pen and a highlighter, and if you are like me, you will also grab some Post-it notes. This book is meant to be your workbook. It is meant to be written in, underlined, doodled in, highlighted, and disfigured—pages bent back and tabbed, and spine broken. This is an active process, and I want you to be involved in it. You may have never done this before because you did not want to ruin or mess up your book, or you wanted to loan the book to another person. Not this time! I want you to set a goal to find at least one new golden nugget of information (something useful that you have discovered and extracted) in each of the four areas of health and wellness, that you can implement immediately. When you find a golden nugget circle it, underline it, star it, or highlight it, so you can find it again. Then, write it down so you remember what you have learned. Notice there are extra blank pages in the back of this book for that very reason. When something sparks an idea in you or you find your key takeaway, write it down on **Worksheet A: Your Golden Nuggets** in the back of the book. I want you to make a reference list of all the best ideas you can get from this book. These nuggets might help you expand your knowledge on the topic, gain a new skill, or broaden your perspective. They might also help you adapt to changes in your future or boost your self-confidence. As we dive into this book, grab those significant points, and let them serve as your coach to guide and train you to live a healthier, more balanced life. This is how you maximize your health and vitality!

EMPOWER yourself through obstacles. Feeling empowered through obstacles refers to the strength, confidence, and self-assurance you experience when facing and overcoming challenges. Whether you like it or not, hurdles will always be a part of your journey. Therefore, you must create a mindset that views these obstacles not as unconquerable barriers, but rather as opportunities for personal growth, learning, and resilience. Empowerment in the face of obstacles often includes developing a positive mindset, recognizing your own ability to achieve your goals, finding inspiration and determination to pursue understanding, managing your emotions, and taking ownership of your own actions and decisions. It is not about avoiding difficulties but embracing them and becoming better at overcoming challenges, despite them.

ENGAGE in environments and associations that help you make deliberate and inspired choices. **There is power in numbers.** Set yourself up for success by attaching yourself to others who want what you want, and desire to see you succeed. Built on trust, respect, and shared goals for success, these meaningful relationships and collaborations work to elevate you. They are key to adding value to each other as you offer your skills, expertise, and assistance to build mutually beneficial relationships. Identify mentors who can provide guidance and support to significantly boost your personal growth. Success is a collective effort, and your network can play a crucial role in your journey. Make it a goal to cultivate your environment.

EXECUTE by creating an action plan. Exceptional execution starts with a vision to narrow your focus. You must clearly identify where you want to go and what you want to accomplish. This is your road map to reaching your short- and long-term goals, tackling hurdles as they arise, revising your path as needed, and reaching successful results. Consistency is key. You must act as if *every day is game day*, and decide it is time to show up for yourself. It is here that you also measure what you manage to stay engaged and motivated, highlight your wins, analyze your failures, course correct as necessary, and create your ultimate vitality management system for success.

ENJOY the journey. The focus of this book is to become a better you, a more balanced you, a more energized you, and a more vitalized you. Do not get so focused on the process that you lose sight of the end goal. Be present in the moment and appreciate the small joys of everyday life. Celebrate the small victories along the way. View challenges as opportunities for growth rather than obstacles for failure. Surround yourself with positivity. Be flexible and embrace spontaneity. **And most importantly... smile, laugh, and have fun!**

A QUICK NOTE ABOUT THIS BOOK

You may find you have enough knowledge of one particular chapter, so you can skip it entirely. The great thing about this book is that you can! Want to dive straight into the food? Read Chapter 4 "Focus on Your Fork" first. Think you already know everything you need to know about exercise? Skip Chapter 6 "Movement is Key" altogether. You will not hurt my feelings. My guess is if you are reading this book right now, you believe you have something to learn. My goal for you is that by the last pages, you have become more mindful, more intentional, and more consistent in balancing your life. I hope you decide what is important and let the rest go. Ask yourself "Does this choice support the lifestyle I am creating?" Find your golden nuggets. It is time for you to have a Yellow Light Moment, so grab your pen and your highlighter and let's get started!

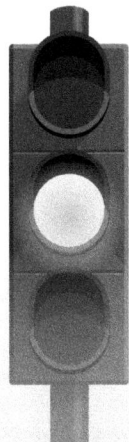

PART I
Evaluate

CHAPTER 1

The Vitality Evaluation

DO YOU FEEL misaligned with your health and wellness? Do you need a moment to recalibrate your vitality? We live in an incredibly fast-paced world, and it is common for us to occasionally need a life audit. I am encouraging you to take a moment to reflect on your vitality to become aware of how you are doing. This is a time for you to stop and evaluate what you are doing so you can become more mindful of your perspective. Not having an accurate perspective can be dangerous at times. Think about the stories you tell yourself and the excuses you make to yourself about your behaviors, in order to make yourself feel better when you do not want to do the things that you know would make you feel healthier. The reality is excuses make today easy, while making tomorrow hard. Discipline makes today hard, but tomorrow easy. You probably rename, justify, or rationalize your habits and actions to make them sound better. For example, when you think that one additional serving of cheesy mashed potatoes at dinner is not that many calories and will not matter because you were active all day. When skipping your workout one more time will not hurt your consistency and reliability. When missing a few hours of sleep really will not affect your productivity, focus, and drive the next day at work. When you do not need self-care because pushing through life is what everyone does to stay at the top of their game. When you say you are "fine" because your troubles are not as bad as someone else's. Self-awareness of your thoughts and actions can catalyze you into change and improvement. Take a moment to look for your own blind spots. These are the areas in which you can fall short of greatness in your life.

SELF-REFLECTION

Self-reflection is the intentional process of diving deep into your thoughts, attitudes, behaviors, emotions, motivations, and desires while determining the "why" behind them. It is taking time to analyze not only how life is going, but how you are responding to different circumstances, situations, and events along the way. It's time to gain perspective and determine whether you're satisfied with the direction your life is heading or if you'd like to adjust to change the outcome. When emotions and opinions can cloud judgment, you can lose sight of the things that truly matter. This is when self-reflection provides clarity and transparency. By improving your ability to be more self-aware, you can better navigate your situations and realities as you learn to manage your thoughts and feelings. Instead of reacting to circumstances that come your way, you can pause and take the time to consider your words, your actions, and the consequences of both.

Without self-reflection, you are simply moving through life without ever taking the time to ask yourself, "Is it going well?" When you don't take the Yellow Light Moments to pause, to analyze, to reconsider, to course correct, to grow, you will end up feeling stuck. You spin on the hamster wheel, repeating the same actions over and over, getting the same results over and over—even if those results are not what you truly desire. Self-reflection can be difficult, and it should not be considered a one-time practice. But in the end, the benefits of practicing self-reflection on a regular basis outweigh the challenge of living a life unexamined.

Self-reflection allows you to look at habits you want to keep, and habits you want to break. Some examples include:

- **Current Habit:** Living a sedentary lifestyle that includes long hours sitting at a desk during the day, and in front of the TV at night, avoiding the need for more physical activity.

Growth Habit: Choosing to set a reminder alarm to stand and move around every hour while at work, and/or beginning a gym routine three days a week before work, so you get it done first thing in the morning.

- **Current Habit:** Grabbing fast food on your way home from work because you are too tired to cook and need to rush back out the door for your night's activities.
Growth Habit: Choosing to grocery shop and meal prep on Sunday so you are prepared for the week with healthy dinner options.

- **Current Habit:** Staying up late at night binging a new series while mindlessly scrolling social media, then finding you are exhausted the next day, leading to a Big Gulp soda in the afternoon to beat the energy slump.
Growth Habit: Choosing to get 7–9 hours of sleep by establishing a consistent sleep routine and creating a sleep-friendly environment where you look forward to climbing into bed.

- **Current Habit:** Not saying "no" to all the extras (the meetings, the committees, the volunteering opportunities, the groups, the events) because you have FOMO (fear of missing out) and guilt from not being involved, leaving you feeling overcommitted and stressed.
Growth Habit: Choosing JOMO (the joy of missing out) as you are learning to stay in and disconnect, keeping yourself feeling charged.

- **Current Habit:** Not drinking enough water throughout the day.
Growth Habit: Choosing to drink half your body weight in ounces every day by setting a timer to drink one bottle of water when you wake up, one bottle by mid-morning, one bottle with lunch, one bottle during your commute home, and one bottle with dinner, limiting your sugary and caffeinated drinks.

- **Current Habit:** Self-sabotaging your health and wellness by focusing on your past failures with change, comparing yourself to your prior self and to others, focusing on things you cannot control, and letting yourself get discouraged with your progress. **Growth Habit:** Choosing to journal your feelings each night before bed focusing on positive affirmations, the amazing things you accomplish every day, and rewriting your narratives.

Feel proud knowing you have developed good habits and ask yourself how you plan to stay on track. When you learn to take a Yellow Light Moment to pause, think, and reflect, you can make improvements and learn from your past experiences. Self-reflection, if done with the true intent of bettering yourself, will lead to positive self-development, self-improvement, and an increase in self-esteem and self-confidence, as you feel more in control of "why" you do the things you do.

THE VITALITY SELF-EVALUATION

Now it is time for you to enter into a time of self-reflection. Start by finding a quiet space, away from distractions, turn off your phone or anything that can disturb you. The goal is to connect with yourself to get an honest reading with how your life is going. Try not to be too harsh with yourself but look for truth in your answers. Remember, no one is the picture of perfection, so don't look for that. Let curiosity be your guide as you allow yourself to dive further into the reasons behind your answers. Consider whether there is a feeling, thought, memory, or belief connected to your answer. Write your answers down to better help you explore your thoughts and feelings. This is a great way to see if there are any patterns or triggers that follow your thoughts and actions.

The first step to having your Yellow Light Moment is to honestly assess your habits and routines. These are your daily practices—I refer to as them as my "dailies."

Take time to genuinely reflect on each one of these questions and write out your answers in **Worksheet B: The Vitality Self-Evaluation** provided at the back of this book, in a notebook, or a journal. Do not rush, or you will miss the value of this self-reflection.

Remember these self-reflection questions are powerful tools you can use to inspire and empower you to discover your health and wellness patterns.

Save your answers, and use these questions to review, readjust, refocus, and recommit to balancing your life every 30–60 days.

Sleep

1. How many hours of sleep do I typically get each night? Am I consistently achieving the recommended 7–9 hours of sleep every night for adults?
2. How alert do I typically feel during the day? Am I relying on caffeine to get me through my morning or afternoon slump, am I having trouble staying awake?
3. Is my bedroom set up as an inviting space to retreat, rest, and rejuvenate? Have I made efforts to create a relaxing bedtime routine?
4. Am I taking naps that are too long or too late in the day that could be affecting my sleep?
5. How many times do I wake up during the night, on average? Are these awakenings brief, or do I find it challenging to return to sleep?
6. Do I wake up feeling refreshed and energized, or do I often feel fatigued?
7. How long does it take me to fall asleep after getting into bed? Am I struggling to fall asleep, and if so, how often?
8. Do I value sleep, or do I feel it is time wasted when I could be accomplishing things?
9. Have I experienced any changes in physical health that may impact my sleep (chronic pain, respiratory issues, etc.)?
10. How would I rate my sleep on a scale of 1–10?

Nutrition

1. Am I feeding myself to fuel my body or am I eating because I am tired, stressed, emotional, bored, or attempting to numb a pain?
2. Is my kitchen organized, clean, and ready to receive and prepare food?
3. Do I have the time in my day and week to prep the food I need to support my work hours, family, exercise, and health issues?
4. If I do not have the time to prep and cook food, do I have a system set in place for quick on-the-go healthy, and delicious meals?

5. How many meals am I cooking at home that are fresh vs. what is ultra-processed or fast food?
6. Is food bringing me joy or do I feel constant guilt and shame around eating?
7. Am I craving sweets, caffeine, salt, and carbs?
8. Am I constantly hungry, or do I wake up hungry in the middle of the night?
9. How much water do I drink during a typical day?
10. How would I rate the quality and quantity of my meals, snacks, and drinks on a scale of 1–10?

Self-Care

1. Do I know the difference between being tired because I need rest, or because I need peace?
2. Am I having mood swings, or do I lack the ability to deal with the day-to-day hurdles that come my way?
3. Am I feeling centered and nurturing my spiritual well-being and connection with my faith during challenging times?
4. Am I setting boundaries so I can take time to recharge myself?
5. Do I need a therapist to help me build tools and skills to weather the harder parts of life?
6. Am I prioritizing self-care, or do I feel guilty for taking a timeout or taking time away from my family, for myself?
7. Do I ever just sit quietly to be alone with my thoughts, or is every minute of my day already scheduled and full of noise?
8. Am I practicing stress-management techniques, such as deep breathing and meditation?
9. Do I maintain heathy relationships and connect regularly with supportive friends and family?
10. How would I rate my stress level on a scale of 1–10?

Movement

1. Am I incorporating 4–5 days of cardio and 2–3 days of strength training each week?
2. Am I completing intentional exercise during my day or am I

counting my regular routine as an activity?
3. Do I find joy in exercising, or does it feel like an obligation?
4. Am I stretching as active recovery after my workouts?
5. Do I need to find ways to mix up my exercise routine (i.e., yoga, swimming, a group fitness class, hiking a new nature trail)?
6. Do I feel confident knowing what I need to do to exercise my body, or do I need to hire a professional to get me started, vary my routines, and keep me accountable?
7. Do I find excuses for why I cannot go to the gym or get regular exercise?
8. Do I find myself socializing at the gym instead of keeping myself accountable for why I am there?
9. Do I truly believe regular exercise is important to my health and should be made a priority?
10. How would I rate my cardiorespiratory endurance, muscular strength, muscular endurance, flexibility, and body composition on a scale of 1–10?

CHAPTER 2

Are You Stable?

THE FOUNDATION of your well-being rests upon the stability of your health. Achieving and maintaining stability in health and wellness is a complex journey that encompasses multiple dimensions, including physical, mental, and emotional health. It is time to look past the absence of illness or injury as a definition of health. Instead, define health as being in a dynamic state of balance that allows you to navigate life with resilience and vitality. Consider that for your health to be stable, it needs to be built on a solid foundation. Many objects built on a solid foundation have a base of four cornerstones. For example, a table, a chair, a bed frame, a car, a dog, or a room. These all have four standard points of contact that play an integral part in providing stability and strength to its overall structure. Consider a table. Depending on how you rearrange the legs under the top of the table, you can take one leg away and still have a functional place to sit and eat, but take one more leg away and you are left trying to balance on the two remaining legs. When discussing your health and wellness, think about them as you would that table. I believe there are four points of contact you need to focus on to maximize your physical, mental, and emotional stability and strength: sleep, nutrition, self-care, and movement. Balancing these four areas is how you build a solid foundation to maximize your health and vitality. Without all four points, you might feel you can still live a balanced life but keep removing points and I bet you start to feel more than a little shaky. Ask yourself, "Am I thriving in my health and wellness?" Everyone experiences moments in their lives when one of these areas is affected and is performing less than optimally. Achieving stability in these areas does not necessarily mean a complete absence of challenges, disturbances, complications, or fluctuations; but rather having the resources and resilience to navigate life's uncertainties without feeling overwhelmed or crashing and returning to a "normal" or "optimal" state. For example, new parents run low on sleep. They are up soothing their baby throughout the night, even knowing they must work the next day. Employees skip their lunch hour and midday meditation as they push to meet strict deadlines at work. Travelers get delayed and are stranded in the airport trying to find a balanced meal while wandering the terminal waiting for their next flight. The workout enthusiast walks out the front door and slips on a patch of ice resulting in an injury that keeps them from hitting the weights for the next 4–6 weeks as they heal. In this chapter, I simply want you to answer the question, "Do I feel stable?" Let me give you a few guidelines to consider:

- Are you getting quality sleep that leaves you feeling fully awake and alert during the day?
- Are you consuming nutritious meals that fuel your body?
- Are you managing the obstacles in your life without major mental, emotional, or physical breakdowns?
- Are you intentionally moving in ways to enhance your cardiovascular and musculoskeletal health?
- Do you feel a sense of overall balance and well-being?

Your degree of health and wellness passes through seasons of life, testing your ability to find balance between all four points—sleep, nutrition, self-care, and movement. One isolated life event is not a game changer, but multiple extended events over time of sleepless nights, not managing your stress, feeding on ultra-processed and high-fat foods, and being sedentary can have an adverse effect on your body. Here's what that can look like:

- energy fades
- craving spikes
- increased headaches
- skin breakouts
- achy and stiff joints
- more frequent mood swings
- poor quality of sleep
- increased heart rate
- inability to focus on the task at hand

Suddenly life is coming at you, and you are not able to cope and respond with a stable and strong body and mind. So, what do you do? Your end goal is not merely to add years to your life, but rather to add health to your years. This is the concept of health span vs. lifespan. You add to your health in what you do daily. Dailies are the small things you do every day that add up over your lifetime.

Over the next four chapters you are invited to take a Yellow Light Moment and assess your health and wellness dailies to maximize your vitality! Realize that simple, consistent changes, in alignment with your goals, can bring real results. Life is a sum of your choices, as illustrated in the figure below. It is time to raise your awareness and enhance your understanding of how daily habits affect your vitality. This will allow you to find solutions for improvement to achieve long-term changes in your life.

FIGURE 2-1: Vitality

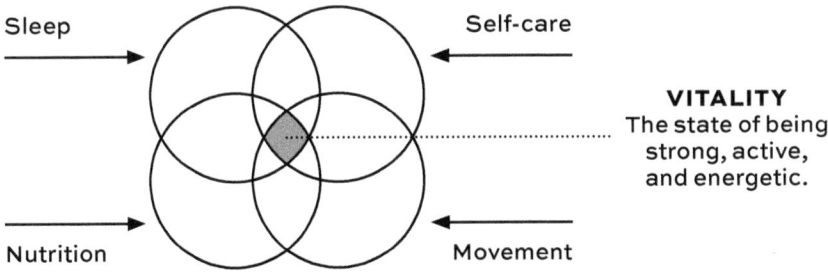

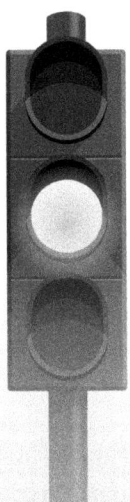

PART II
Educate

CHAPTER 3

Find Your Zzzs

SLEEP is incredibly important for your health. Without it, you are not performing with optimum efficiency. Though sleep needs vary from person to person, most adults require between 7 and 9 hours of quality sleep per night. Yet, up to 35 percent of adults in the United States do not get enough sleep.[1] Think of sleep as a giant reset button for your physical, emotional, and mental health. Over time, lack of sleep is associated with multiple negative health effects. Consider that poor sleep is linked to having:

- an impaired immune function
- disruption in hormones
- increased risk of heart disease
- increased and elevated blood pressure
- increased risk of developing type 2 diabetes and insulin resistance
- increased inflammation with activated inflammatory signaling
- higher risk of metabolic syndrome
- increased depression
- decreased motivation for exercise
- decreased cognition
- decreased concentration

- decreased productivity
- decreased performance
- decreased reaction time
- reduction in ability to regulate emotions, interact socially, and show empathy

Sleep gives your body, including your brain, time to repair itself and conduct important functions. While you are sleeping, your brain stores new information and gets rid of toxic waste. Nerve cells communicate and reorganize, supporting healthy brain function. The body repairs cells, restores energy, and releases molecules, like hormones and proteins. When you do not get good sleep, or you sleep fewer than seven hours per night, you fall into a cascade of results that do not always benefit you. Take into consideration how lack of sleep is associated with an increased risk of weight gain. Sleep deprivation may increase your appetite and cause you to eat more calories, increasing levels of ghrelin and decreasing levels of leptin.[2] Ghrelin, often referred to as the "hunger hormone," signals the brain to initiate eating. Leptin, often referred to as the "satiety hormone," signals fullness to the brain helping regulate appetite and food intake. Lack of sleep may also result in a lack of motivation to go to the gym, hit the trails, or whatever exercise you choose because you are more tired. Chronic sleep deprivation is associated with an increased risk of heart disease, high blood pressure, and stroke. It's during sleep that your heart rate and blood pressure lower, giving your cardiovascular system a much-needed break. Lack of sleep is closely linked to mood swings, irritability, and increased stress levels. When you are well-rested, you're better equipped to handle life's challenges with a more positive outlook.

---

[1] Liu, Y., Wheaton, A. G., Chapman, D. P., Cunningham, T. J., Lu, H., & Croft, J. B. (2016). Prevalence of healthy sleep duration among adults–United States, 2014. Morbidity and Mortality Weekly Report, 65(6), 137–141., Retrieved March 24, 2023, from https://pubmed.ncbi.nlm.nih.gov/26890214/

[2] Schmid SM, Hallschmid M, Jauch-Chara K, Born J, Schultes B. A single night of sleep deprivation increases ghrelin levels and feelings of hunger in normal-weight healthy men. J Sleep Res. 2008 Sep;17(3):331-4. doi: 10.1111/j.1365-2869.2008.00662.x. Epub 2008 Jun 28. PMID: 18564298.

THE ANATOMY OF SLEEP

While it is normal to think about how many hours you sleep every night, it is also crucial to consider whether you are getting restorative sleep during those hours. What, therefore, constitutes a good night's sleep? Sleep is divided into cycles and stages. In a typical night, a person experiences four to six sleep cycles.[3] Not all of these sleep cycles are the same length during the night, but on average they last about 90 minutes each. Many variables can affect your sleep cycles—alcohol consumption, medications, sleep disorders, recent sleep patterns, and age.

In a normal sleep cycle, there are four sleep stages. Each of these stages plays a role in your mind and body waking up and feeling refreshed and rejuvenated the next day. The first three stages are non-rapid eye movement sleep, also known as non-REM or NREM sleep. The fourth stage is rapid eye movement sleep or REM sleep. When you first fall asleep and your body enters light sleep, you are in NREM Stage 1, also called N1. During this stage your brain waves, heart rate, and eye movements slow down while your muscles start to relax. It is easy to wake someone up during this stage but if left undisturbed they will enter stage 2. This stage normally lasts from one to seven minutes.[4] During NREM Stage 2, or N2, your heartbeat and breathing slow down even further. There are no eye moments, your body temperature drops, and your brain activity slows. You can be awakened easily during this stage of sleep which can last for 10–25 minutes during the first sleep cycle. Afterward, each N2 stage can become longer during the night.[4] The third stage of non-REM sleep is the deepest sleep stage called NREM Stage 3, or N3. In this stage your body performs a variety of important health promoting tasks. Your heartbeat and breathing are now at their slowest rate. There are no eye movements, your body is fully relaxed, your immune system strengthens, your tissues repair and grow, and cell regeneration

---

[3] Patel AK, Reddy V, Shumway KR, et al. Physiology, Sleep Stages. [Updated 2022 Sep 7]. In: StatPearls [Internet]. Treasure Island (FL): StatPearls Publishing; 2023 Jan-. Available from: https://www.ncbi.nlm.nih.gov/books/NBK526132/

[4] Kirsch, D. (2021, November 8). Stages and architecture of normal sleep. In A.F. Eichler (Ed.). UpToDate., Retrieved December 6, 2022, from https://www.uptodate.com/contents/stages-and-architecture-of-normal-sleep

occurs. It is harder to wake someone up in N3, which commonly lasts for about 20–40 minutes. NREM stages shorten as you continue sleeping, and more time is instead spent in REM sleep.

REM sleep is the final stage of sleep (rapid eye movement sleep). This is the stage where eye movements become rapid (hence the name of this stage), and your breathing and heart rate increase and become more varied. Limb muscles become temporarily paralyzed as the body experiences atonia (a deficiency of muscle tone), brain activity markedly increases, and most of your dreaming occurs. REM sleep is believed to be essential to cognitive functions like memory,[4] learning, and creativity.[5] Under normal circumstances, you do not enter REM sleep stage until you have been asleep for about 90 minutes. As the night goes on, REM stages lengthen, especially during the second half of the night. In total, REM stages make up around 25 percent of sleep in adults.[6]

PRIORITIZE YOUR SLEEP

Rest is often the first thing that is sacrificed when life gets busy. We wear ourselves out with the frantic pace of life and the goal of "getting it all done." Many people fail to find the importance of having a quality sleep hygiene routine. How many people unplug by plugging in? It's easy to overlook the value of sleep and instead exchange your rest time for— scrolling social media, working a few extra hours, staying out socializing, and binging the newest streaming series. Perhaps you *survive* on 4-6 hours of sleep when you could *thrive* on 7–9 hours of quality sleep. When you evaluate the quality of your sleep, there are different categories to consider. I want you to assess the duration of your sleep, the onset of your sleep or how difficult it is for you to fall asleep, the continuity of your sleep, the

---

[5] Cai, D. J., Mednick, S. A., Harrison, E. M., Kanady, J. C., & Mednick, S. C. (2009). REM, not incubation, improves creativity by priming associative networks. Proceedings of the National Academy of Sciences of the United States of America, 106(25), 10130–10134. https://pubmed.ncbi.nlm.nih.gov/19506253/

[6] Suni, Eric, and Singh, Dr. Abhinav. (2023, December 8). Stages of sleep: what happens in a sleep cycle. Sleep Foundation.org https://www.sleepfoundation.org//stages-of-sleep

quality of your sleep, and the environment where you sleep. Also weigh your daytime alertness, the use of sleep aids, and your physical health related to your sleep. The questions you answered in the Vitality Evaluation will help you assess various aspects of your sleep and provide valuable insights into potential areas for improvement.

How much sleep do *you* need? The amount of sleep each person needs will vary, but the National Sleep Foundation recommends at least:[7]

- 14–17 hours for newborns (0–3 months)
- 12–15 hours for infants (4–11 months)
- 11–14 hours for 1- and 2-year-olds
- 10–13 hours for 3- to 5-year-olds
- 9–11 hours for 6- to 13-year-olds
- 8–10 hours for 14- to 17-year-olds
- 7–9 hours for adults
- 7–8 hours for adults 65 and older

Making sleep a priority takes a few conscious decisions. It is time to find your golden nuggets to maximize your sleep.

Create a Bedroom Experience

Your bedroom should be an environment that reduces your stress, decreases your stimuli, and invites you to escape into restful slumber. Remember that everyone's preferences are different, so it is important to customize these suggestions to your own needs and preferences by experimenting with different elements for the best results. Think **quiet, dark, cool, cozy,** and **calm.**

---

[7] Max Hirshkowitz, Kaitlyn Whiton, Steven M. Albert, Cathy Alessi, Oliviero Bruni, Lydia DonCarlos, Nancy Hazen, John Herman, Eliot S. Katz, Leila Kheirandish-Gozal, David N. Neubauer, Anne E. O'Donnell, Maurice Ohayon, John Peever, Robert Rawding, Ramesh C. Sachdeva, Belinda Setters, Michael V. Vitiello, J. Catesby Ware, Paula J. Adams Hillard. National Sleep Foundation's sleep time duration recommendations: methodology and results summary. Sleep Health, Volume 1, Issue 1. 2015, ISSN 2352-7218, https://doi.org/10.1016/j.sleh.2014.12.010.

- **Quiet.** Unexpected noises can disrupt you during shallower sleep cycles and interfere with your quality of sleep. Minimize sound by creating a soft barrier—utilizing a fan or white noise machine. Adding a thick rug and heavy blinds will also help buffer noises and contribute to a more peaceful sleep environment.
- **Dark.** Your body is programmed to sleep when it is dark, as light inhibits the production of melatonin. Dim the lights while getting ready for bed and decrease the light in your room with room-darkening shades or dark curtains.
- **Cool.** Your body temperature naturally drops as you drift off to sleep. Turn the thermostat down at least 5–10 degrees to achieve a cooler temperature in the bedroom, or sleep with lighter blankets. A bedroom between 60–67 degrees Fahrenheit tells your body it is time to snooze.
- **Cozy.** Add an element of comfort with high-quality bedding, including pillows, sheets, and blankets that makes you feel pampered. Try incorporating a weighted blanket, something with texture, or a color that soothes you. Opt for fabrics like cotton or linen for a breathable and relaxed feel on your skin. This might also be an appropriate time to invest in a comfortable mattress that supports your sleeping posture. The right support can make a significant difference in the quality of your sleep. If you often have cold feet when you climb into bed, start with wearing a warm pair of socks, or place an electric blanket at the foot of your bed to warm them up.
- **Calm.** Get rid of anything in your bedroom that distracts you from sleep. This means no treadmill, computer, piles of laundry, or reminders of tomorrow's tasks. Create a space that eases your mind and reduces your stress. Remember: bedrooms are for sleeping not working. Use calming scents, such as lavender, chamomile, or cedarwood—in essential oils or diffusers. These scents are known to have a relaxing effect on the mind and body. Try adding a few drops of essential oil to a cotton ball near your bed at night. Personalize your space by adding individual touches to your bedroom that bring you joy—such as photos or

artwork. An intimate space can create a sense of comfort and relaxation.

Remember, your bedroom should be a sanctuary—a place where you can unwind, relax, and drift off into restorative sleep. By engineering your sleep environment to cater to your preferences and needs, you're setting the stage for deep, rejuvenating rest each night.

Regarding the quality of your sleep environment: Sometimes "who" we sleep with can be a sleep disrupter. This may be a significant other or a pet, and it is okay to have an honest conversation if part of your sleep problem is that you sleep better alone. If your sleep partner snores, sleeps with a CPAP machine, creates extra body heat, has a different sleep pattern because of their occupation, talks in their sleep, moves or kicks excessively, or any number of other sleep-disrupting patterns to you, it is a good time to evaluate if sleeping separately is more beneficial to your overall health. It should not bring feelings of guilt, failure, separation, or anxiety. Sleeping alone can be a healthy choice as it allows you to create an optimal sleep environment tailed to your individual needs, leading to better quality rest and overall well-being.

Stick to a Schedule

Consistency is the key to life, and this is especially true when it comes to sleep. The body has a natural internal clock known as the circadian rhythm, which regulates the sleep-wake cycle. When you follow a sleep schedule by going to bed and waking up at the same time each day, your body becomes familiar with a particular sleep routine, making it easier to fall asleep and stay asleep in turn promoting better quality sleep. When in doubt, set an alarm that reminds you it is time to start winding down at night instead of looking at the clock wondering where the night has gone. And yes, that includes staying consistent on the weekends and vacations.

Reduce Blue Light

Blue light, especially the kind emitted by electronic devices such as smartphones, tablets, and computers, can stimulate your body to produce cortisol, a daytime hormone, while also suppressing the production of melatonin. For this reason, decrease your exposure to blue light 60–90 minutes before bed. Exposing yourself to blue light in the evening can delay the onset of sleep. Additionally, prolonged exposure to screens can cause eye strain and discomfort. If you must use a device at night, consider using blue blocker glasses. These glasses are designed to filter out or block a portion of the blue light emitted from digital screens and artificial light sources.

PG Your Night

Viewing or listening to violent or disturbing forms of media before bedtime can stir up strong emotions such as fear, stress, anxiety, or anger, which can interfere with the body's ability to relax and transition into restful sleep. The emotional impact of disturbing content can linger even after you have turned off the screen, making it harder to achieve a calm and positive mindset beneficial to sleep, while increasing the likelihood of experiencing nightmares. In addition, exposure to blue light, common in electronic devices, can also interfere with the body's natural circadian rhythms. Try to engage in calming activities before bedtime, such as reading a light book, practicing relaxation techniques, listening to soothing music, and keeping your conversations light before bed.

Time Your Naps

Timing your naps is important because it can significantly affect the benefits you receive from the nap and your overall sleep-wake cycle. There are a few key factors to consider when timing your naps. First, consider the sleep stages. NREM sleep is the initial stage of sleep where you are not dreaming. Napping for about 20–30 minutes allows you to stay in this stage, helping with alertness and performance without experiencing sleep inertia, that groggy feeling after waking up. REM sleep occurs in longer naps that last around 60–90 minutes. This sleep stage is crucial for memory consolidation and creativity. Waking during REM can lead to feeling dazed. Completing the full REM cycle provides more profound benefits. Next, remember your body has natural rhythms that influence alertness and drowsiness at various times of the day. The ideal time for a nap is in the early afternoon, between 2 p.m. and 3 p.m. as it follows the post-lunch dip in alertness. Napping too close to bedtime may interfere with your ability to fall asleep at night, therefore, it is generally recommended to avoid napping in the late afternoon or evening. Finally, consistency in nap timing can help regulate your circadian rhythm and improve overall sleep quality. If you nap at the same time each day, your body may become accustomed to the routine.

Cut Off Caffeine

As a central nervous system stimulant, caffeine can disrupt your natural sleep-wake cycle by blocking adenosine receptors in the brain. Adenosine is a neurotransmitter that promotes sleep and relaxation, therefore, interfering with it can disturb the normal progression of sleep. According to the American Academy of Sleep Medicine, caffeine's half-life is up to 5 hours, which is the amount of time it takes for a quantity of a substance to be reduced to half of the original amount.[8] This means if you consume 100 milligrams of caffeine, at 3–5 hours, there could still be approximately 50 milligrams of caffeine remaining in your system. So that late afternoon caffeine break could hinder your sleep, depending on when you turn the lights out. There are additional individual factors to consider such as age, liver function, pregnancy, and certain medications that can affect how quickly the body metabolizes caffeine. Additionally, sensitivity to caffeine can vary among individuals. Some people may feel the effects of caffeine for shorter or longer durations. To optimize sleep hygiene, avoid consuming caffeine, or at least limit its intake, in the hours leading up to bed.

Exercise Regularly

Exercise can have both positive and negative effects on sleep—depending on several factors such as timing and intensity. People who engage in regular exercise often report experiencing deeper and more restorative sleep. Exercise is an effective stress reliever and helps regulate the circadian rhythm when done at the same time each day. Try not to work out too late

---

[8] American Academy of Sleep Medicine. (29 January, 2018) Sleep and Caffeine. http://sleepeducation.org/sleep-caffeine.

in the day, but rather 2–4 hours before bedtime to give your body enough time to efficiently cool down. If you are nearing bedtime and feel the need to move but you know it tends to keep you awake, try slow-paced yoga or stretching.

Stop Eating 2–3 Hours Before Bedtime

Different foods, when they are digested, affect the body in various ways. While some foods can cause bloating and indigestion, others may contribute to acid reflux or cause a fluctuation in blood sugar. All these situations can result in restlessness and wakefulness during the night. For these reasons, if you are hungry close to bedtime, consider having a light and easy-to-digest snack under 250 calories that is low in sugar and caffeine. Preferable snacks include a tablespoon of peanut butter on whole grain toast, a bowl of oats with blueberries, a handful of nuts (almonds, walnuts, pistachios, cashews), tuna on cucumber slices, kiwi, avocado toast, spinach and eggs, or tart cherries or cherry juice.

Cut Off Alcohol

Stop drinking alcohol at least three hours before bedtime. Although alcohol may initially make you feel drowsy and help you fall asleep faster, its impact on sleep is more complex and can have negative consequences. Remember REM sleep is a crucial stage of the sleep cycle associated with dreaming and memory consolidation. Alcohol consumption has been linked to a reduction in REM sleep, potentially affecting your cognitive function and mood. Furthermore, as alcohol is metabolized in the body, it can lead to an increase in wakefulness during the second half of the night, disrupting the natural sleep cycle. Alcohol also has a muscle-relaxing effect which includes the muscles in the throat. This relaxation can exacerbate snoring and increase the risk of sleep apnea, a condition where breathing temporarily stops during sleep. Additionally, alcohol is a diuretic, meaning it can increase urine production and lead to more frequent trips to the bathroom during the night, disrupting sleep and contributing to dehydration. It is important to note that individual responses to alcohol can vary, and factors such as the amount of alcohol consumed, the timing of consumption, and individual differences in metabolism play a role.

Do Not Stay in Bed if You Cannot Sleep
It is ideal to break the association between the bed and wakefulness. If you have been in bed tossing and turning for more than 20–30 minutes, do not continue to lie there. By lying in bed awake for an extended period, your brain may start to associate the bed with being awake, making it more difficult to fall asleep when you do lie down. Staying in bed while being unable to sleep can also lead to increased anxiety and frustration. This anxiety can further disrupt your ability to relax and fall asleep. Getting out of bed and engaging in a quiet, relaxing activity can help reduce this anxiety. Try doing some light stretching, journaling, reading a short article, walking around the house, or meditating. Just remember—no blue lights! Do not grab your phone, tablet, computer, or turn on the TV.

Intentionally Wind Down
There are numerous practices that support closing out your day to transition you to sleep. As you explore these options, stay open minded regarding incorporating any of them into your routine, knowing different people need different things at different stages of life.

- **Empty your brain.** Emptying your brain before bed refers to the practice of clearing your mind and reducing mental clutter to promote better sleep and relaxation. If your mind tends to race as soon as you close your eyes at night, then keep a pen and paper next to your bed to jot down your late-night ideas, worries, and tasks for the next day. This helps externalize your thoughts and can be a way of mentally letting go.
- **Make a to-do list.** Create a to-do list for the next day to help organize your tasks and manage your time. Knowing you have a plan can help alleviate the anxiety of forgetting important tasks. Consider using productivity apps or tools that allow you to set reminders and synchronize your to-do list across devices. As you are prioritizing your list, decide if you would rather begin with an easy, quick task to kick off your day, helping you feel accomplished, or if you want to tackle the hardest item on your list to get it out of the way. Throughout your day, regularly review

your list, cross off completed tasks, and reassess priorities if necessary.
- **Meditate.** This is a practice of mindfulness that encourages you to calm your mind. These mental exercises are known to increase relaxation and reduce stress. This can be particularly helpful before bedtime, as it promotes a more peaceful, clear, and stable state of mind as you transition from external stressors to internal awareness.
- **Gratitude journal.** Expressing your appreciation and thanks for what you have leads to positive emotions in life. When starting a gratitude journal, begin by finding a calming environment and location to help you wind down before bedtime. Select a journal that resonates with you. You may also use a digital journaling app if you prefer. Take a few moments to reflect on your day recalling both the positive and challenging moments you experienced. List three to five things for which you are grateful. These can be simple or significant, ranging from personal achievements to moments of joy, connections with others, or aspects of your life that you often take for granted. Provide details about each gratitude point and elaborate **why** you are grateful for each one, adding depth to your reflections. As you write, try to evoke the emotions associated with each entry. Reflect on how these aspects of your life make you feel blessed, happy, or fulfilled. Occasionally, go back and reread your entries. Reflect on the patterns of gratitude in your life and how your mindset may be changing over time. As you become more accustomed to recognizing and appreciating positive aspects of your life, you may find that your overall outlook eventually becomes more optimistic. Remember, the goal of a gratitude journal is not just to list things but to cultivate a genuine sense of appreciation for the positive aspects of your life.
- **Prayer.** For many people, prayer serves as a profound connection with a higher power, seeking guidance, expressing gratitude, and finding solace. Bedtime can be a time when worries and anxieties surface. Prayer offers an opportunity for you to express concerns and release your burdens while experiencing peace and hope.

This sacred conversation can provide a sense of comfort, security, and calmness. The focused and meditative nature of prayer before sleep can serve as a comforting ritual, helping to quiet the mind, release worries, and invite a sense of divine presence that promotes restful sleep.
- **Deep breathing.** Practice deep breathing exercises to help relax your body and mind. Deep breathing is a simple, yet effective technique that can help release the tension in your body and alleviate stress. When you engage in deep breathing exercises, several physiological responses occur, contributing to a sense of calm and relaxation which helps you to fall asleep. Deep breathing stimulates the parasympathetic nervous system (PNS), which is responsible for the "rest and digest" response. This system counteracts the sympathetic nervous system, which triggers the "fight or flight" response. Activating the PNS promotes relaxation and a reduction in stress. Deep breathing has also been shown to lower cortisol levels—a stress hormone that, when elevated, can contribute to feelings of anxiety and tension. Deep, slow breathing can help regulate your heart rate and blood pressure. This can be particularly helpful in stressful situations where these physiological responses may be heightened.
- **Guided imagery.** Try some visualizations by picturing a peaceful and calming scene in your mind. This mental imagery can help shift your focus away from stressors and promote relaxation, reducing your overall level of stress and anxiety. This mindfulness practice can also help quiet a busy mind and alleviate racing thoughts that may interfere with quality sleep. Guided imagery often includes relaxation exercises, which can help release physical tension in the body. Progressive muscle relaxation, for example, involves tensing and then releasing different muscle groups, promoting a sense of overall physical relaxation.

Don't Snooze

Stop hitting the snooze button. When you go in and out of sleep, it worsens your sleep inertia—the groggy feeling that comes from jolting yourself out of sleep. The fragmented sleep obtained through snoozing is generally of lower quality compared to continuous sleep. Remember, you are trying to establish healthy sleep routines. Going to bed and waking up at the same time every day helps regulate your body's internal clock. Snoozing disrupts this routine and can make it more challenging to establish a consistent sleep pattern. When you rise after that first alarm, you are developing discipline and mental toughness. Resisting the temptation to hit the snooze button requires self-mastery. Building on this trait can positively impact other areas of your life where self-control is important. Breaking the snooze-button habit may take time and effort, but the long-term benefits for your physical and mental health, as well as your productivity, make it a worthwhile goal.

Other Options

Consider familiarizing yourself with non-pharmaceuticals such as herbal supplements, teas, aromatherapy, and bath soaks. Remember to always consult your healthcare professional before starting any new supplement regimen, especially if you are taking medications or have pre-existing health conditions. Your practitioner can provide guidance based on your specific situation and health history. Here are some commonly suggested supplements that may help promote better sleep:

- **Melatonin** is a hormone produced by the pineal gland in your brain and is responsible for regulating your body's circadian rhythm to manage your natural sleep cycle. The production and release of melatonin is influenced by the time of day, with levels typically increasing in the evening as it gets dark, and decreasing in the morning when it gets light.
- **Magnesium** is a mineral involved in over 300 biochemical reactions in the body, including muscle and nerve function. It is found in many foods, including green leafy vegetables, nuts, seeds, and whole grains. Some people find that magnesium supplements can help with relaxation and improve sleep quality.
- **Lavender** refers to a group of plants in the genus Lavandula known for their fragrant flowers and aromatic foliage. These

plants are widely cultivated for their use in various products including perfumes, essential oils, and herbal teas. Lavender oil may have a calming effect, promoting relaxation and better quality of sleep.
- **Valerian root** is an herb that has been used for centuries to treat various ailments, such as anxiety, nervousness, restlessness, and sleep disorders. It may help improve sleep quality and reduce the time it takes to fall asleep.
- **Glycine** is an amino acid that has been studied for its involvement in various metabolic pathways, including the synthesis of nucleic acids and the conversion of glucose into energy. It may help you feel less fatigued during the day.
- **5-HTP (5-Hydroxytryptophan)** is a precursor to serotonin. Serotonin is a neurotransmitter, a chemical messenger that transmits signals to the brain, which can be converted to melatonin. It plays a role in regulating depression, anxiety, and insomnia and is produced in the body from the amino acid tryptophan.
- **L-Theanine** is an amino acid that is commonly found in tea leaves, particularly in green tea. L-Theanine is known for its calming and relaxing effects and is often used as a supplement to promote relaxation, without causing drowsiness.
- **CBD (Cannabidiol)** is a chemical compound found in the Cannabis sativa plant. Available in various forms, including oils, tinctures, capsules, gummies, and topical products; CBD plays a role in regulating various physiological processes, including mood, appetite, and sleep, while also having potential therapeutic benefits such as reducing anxiety, alleviating pain, decreasing inflammation, and improving sleep.

Feed Your Sleep

Certain foods contain compounds that may promote better sleep by influencing the production of sleep-inducing hormones or by providing nutrients that support relaxation. Here are some foods that might help improve your sleep:

- **Turkey** contains tryptophan, an amino acid that can contribute to the production of serotonin and melatonin, both of which are associated with sleep.
- **Salmon, mackerel, and other fatty fish** are rich in omega-3 fatty acids which have been linked to improved sleep quality.
- **Almonds, walnuts, flax seeds, and chia seeds** are reliable sources of magnesium and tryptophan, promoting relaxation and sleep.
- **Bananas** contain tryptophan, potassium, and magnesium, which can help relax muscles.
- **Cherries**, especially tart cherries, are a natural source of melatonin, a hormone that regulates sleep-wake cycles.
- **Oats** are a good source of complex carbohydrates and may help increase the availability of tryptophan in the bloodstream.
- **Dairy products**, such as yogurt, contain calcium, which is involved in the production of melatonin. Greek yogurt is also rich in protein.
- **Chamomile, valerian root, and lavender teas** are known for their calming properties and may help relax the body before bedtime.
- **Kiwi** is rich in serotonin precursors and antioxidants. Because of this some studies suggest that eating kiwi before bed may improve sleep quality.
- **Brown rice, quinoa, and whole wheat bread** provide a good source of complex carbohydrates, which can increase serotonin levels.
- **Dark chocolate** contains small amounts of caffeine, but it is also a source of serotonin precursors. Enjoy it in moderation.
- **A small amount of honey** before bedtime may promote the release of melatonin and help improve sleep quality.

Remember to avoid heavy meals close to bedtime, and know that individual responses to food can vary, so it is a good idea to pay attention to how different foods affect your sleep. Adjust your diet accordingly.

Consider Sleep Disorders

Contemplate if poor and insufficient sleep could be caused by a sleep disorder. It is important to see a sleep specialist when you experience persistent and significant sleep related issues that impact your daily life and well-being. Some situations that may warrant a visit to a sleep specialist include:

- **Chronic insomnia:** You may suffer from this if you have trouble falling asleep or staying asleep on a regular basis, for more than a few weeks, despite making efforts to improve your sleep hygiene.
- **Excessive daytime sleepiness:** If you consistently feel overly tired during the day, regardless of how much you sleep at night, it could be a sign of a sleep disorder.
- **Sleep apnea:** Symptoms such as loud snoring, choking, or gasping during sleep, or frequent awakenings with a sensation of shortness of breath may indicate sleep apnea, a serious condition that requires medical attention.
- **Restless leg syndrome (RLS):** If you experience an irresistible urge to move your legs, especially at night, interfering with your ability to fall asleep, you may have RLS.
- **Narcolepsy:** Characterized by sudden and uncontrollable episodes of falling asleep during the day, or you experience muscle weakness (cataplexy) triggered by strong emotions.
- **Parasomnia:** Engaging in unusual behaviors during sleep, such as sleepwalking, night terrors, or REM behavior disorder.
- **Shift work sleep disorder:** If your work schedule requires you to be awake and active during the night, it may lead to difficulty sleeping during the day.
- **Persistent snoring:** While occasional snoring is common, persistent loud snoring may be a sign of an underlying sleep disorder, such as sleep apnea.
- **Difficulty falling asleep or staying asleep:** If you consistently have trouble initiating or maintaining sleep, it could be a sign of various sleep disorders.
- **Circadian rhythm disorders:** This includes disruptions to your natural sleep-wake cycle, leading to difficulties adjusting to a regular sleep schedule.

If you notice any of these symptoms or have concerns about your sleep, it is advisable to consult with a healthcare professional, such as a primary care physician, who may refer you to a sleep specialist for further evaluation and diagnosis. A sleep specialist can conduct a comprehensive assessment, which may involve a sleep study (polysomnography) or other diagnostic tests to identify the underlying cause of your sleep issues.

Taking care of your sleep is one of the foundations for maximizing your health and vitality. Just like you prioritize your diet, physical activity, and self-care, it is time to give sleep the attention it deserves.

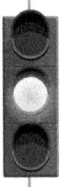

YELLOW LIGHT MOMENT

Turn to **Worksheet C**. It is time for your Yellow Light Moment. Ask yourself:

- How can I optimize my sleep routine?
- What golden nuggets did I take away from this chapter?
- What can I start to implement immediately to improve the quality and quantity of my sleep?

Write 3 action steps and start to implement at least 1 of them this week.

CHAPTER 4

Focus On Your Fork

THE GOAL of this chapter is to do it justice without overwhelming you. Discussing nutrition is a complex task. Let's keep it simple and stick to the basics. My goal is to increase your mindfulness of nutrition with some easily applicable steps to help you improve how you look at food. I also want to help you become more intentional when shopping for it, ordering it, and preparing it. Ultimately ask yourself, "Does this choice support the lifestyle I am creating?" If you want to go beyond the basics of this chapter, I encourage you to talk to your doctor or a registered dietitian for a personalized program that will take into consideration your health status, lifestyle, and food preferences. I know you may simply want me to tell you what I think the ideal diet is. Well, without complicating things or addressing any medical issues, diseases, dietary restrictions, and/or allergies, an excellent diet consists of moderation, eating more protein and veggies than you probably do, increasing your healthy fats and fiber, decreasing sugar and ultra-processed foods, watching your portions, eating slowly and stopping before you are full, drinking lots of water, and occasionally splurging on a dessert or drink to enjoy life. But because I know you want more than that, I am going to break this chapter down into my basics on how to Focus on Your Fork.

FOCUS ON YOUR FORK

"Healthy eating" means fueling your body with nutritious foods. This is not a one-size-fits all concept as the specifics differ for each person based on factors such as age, sex, activity level, and health conditions. Instead, focusing on nutrient-rich foods is the basis of every good plan. Take into consideration the *quantity* and *quality* of the foods you consume but ultimately "quality," aka nutrient-dense foods, are the primary concern. Understand all foods contain calories, but not all foods are nutrient dense. For example, a candy bar or a serving of pasta may be rich in calories, but deficient in essential nutrients such as vitamins, minerals, protein, and fiber. Likewise, items labeled as low-calorie or diet-friendly may have minimal calories but lack nutritional value, so you are getting the calories but missing the nutrients. Let's dig into how you can focus on what you're putting in your body.

Prioritize It

The first step to focusing on your fork is to make food one of your priorities. Making food a priority means giving it a higher level of importance, attention, and focus compared to other tasks, and activities. This is where many of us fall short. When you prioritize your food, you are consciously choosing to allocate your resources—time, money, energy, and effort—to ensure you consume well-balanced, healthy, calorically appropriate meals and snacks. If you have a particularly busy lifestyle, then this means you are prioritizing *whole foods* over quick, easy-to-grab, last-minute fast foods, ultra-processed, and refined options. *Whole foods* refer to foods that are in their natural, unprocessed state or minimally processed to retain most of their original nutritional content. Think fruits, veggies, whole grains, legumes, nuts, seeds, and lean proteins (Tip: shop the perimeter of the grocery store and try to eat seasonally and locally to get fresher options). Whole foods are often more filling than ultra-processed options, which can help curb cravings and reduce your overall calorie intake. Your body will not be sculpted by starvation. It will be created with proper nutrition. It is a journey that starts first in your head by making it a priority.

Read It
Nutrition fact labels provide valuable information about nutritional content and ingredients. By reading a label, you can learn what the recommended serving size is for the food item. The label will also show the percent daily value (%DV) which is the recommended daily intake of the nutrients provided by one serving of the food, based on a daily intake of 2,000 calories. Various nutrients will be listed—including total fat, saturated fat, trans fat, cholesterol, sodium, total carbohydrates, dietary fiber, sugars, and protein. An ingredient list will provide all the ingredients present in the product, usually in descending order by weight. Ingredients with the highest quantity are listed first. The label will also highlight the presence of common allergens such as nuts, milk, eggs, soy, wheat, among others. For individuals with food allergies or intolerances, reading labels is essential to avoid consuming substances that may cause an adverse reaction. An expiration date or best by date will also be present on the label indicating the date by which the product is expected to remain fresh and safe to consume. Understanding how to read labels is a great tool when making informed decisions about your diet and how to manage your intake of specific ingredients. Labels enable consumers to compare various products and choose the one that best aligns with their nutritional needs and preferences.

Track It
Food tracking helps increase your awareness of the total number and type of calories you consume. This awareness is beneficial for maintaining a healthy weight and/or achieving specific fitness goals. Most individuals underestimate the number of calories they eat and drink daily, therefore, tracking is key to providing a more accurate picture. The goal is: Do not eat too little and do not eat too much. By starving yourself, you are restricting your body from vital nutrients and minerals, resulting in lower energy levels. With less energy you may not have the same drive and determination to work out. Eating too little can also slow down your metabolism. Those who skip meals also tend to overeat at subsequent meals, ending with a surplus of calories and a struggle with fluctuating blood sugar levels. On the other side, you could be eating too much. Even if you are eating healthy

foods and getting regular exercise, it is still possible to have too much of a good thing. Sometimes grabbing that quick snack here and there, even when it is a "healthy snack," can pack on an additional 500–900 calories by the end of the day. For example, imagine you walk by a bowl of almonds and grab a handful as a "smart" snack instead of reaching for a handful of candy. You have chosen well. But walk by that bowl three times and you have just added approximately 510 calories. Walk by five times and now you have added 850 extra calories. Even the healthy snacks add up calorically by the end of the day. Using tools like measuring cups, food scales, and food diaries can help you monitor your calorie intake and stay on track. There are also easy-to-use, free apps available to simplify this task.

Tracking not only allows you to monitor total calories but also the type of calories, such as the distribution of macronutrients (carbohydrates, proteins, and fats) and micronutrients (vitamins and minerals). If you have specific health or fitness goals, such as weight loss, muscle gain, or are managing a medical condition, tracking your food can help you set realistic targets and track your progress. It is important to measure this information so you can manage it. Food tracking can also reveal patterns in your eating habits, helping you identify triggers for overeating and making unhealthy choices. This self-awareness is essential for making positive changes. My personal favorite is how tracking creates a sense of accountability. Knowing that you must log everything you eat and drink will most likely influence your food and beverage choices and encourage healthier habits. Let's be honest. There is a moment before you put that next helping of mac 'n cheese on your plate or when you grab the next handful of trail mix or bite-sized chocolate when you stop and think, "If I eat this, I have to track it." Sometimes that thought is enough of a deterrent to walk away and make a better choice. Tracking your food is also very educational. It will help you understand the nutritional content of different foods, promoting informed decision making when it comes to your diet. Knowledge is power. I once had a client come to the realization that not all chicken is created equal. A grilled piece of skinless chicken breast is different from ordering hot wings. These "aha moments" are what I am wanting you to discover. Whether you are an individual with medical conditions, such as diabetes, tracking food to manage blood sugar levels; or an athlete focused on performance to ensure you are fueling your body optimally for physical activities, tracking is a helpful tool. It is important to approach tracking with a balanced mindset and not let it lead to obsessive behaviors. Use it as a tool for self-improvement and not a source of stress or anxiety. Turn to **Worksheet D: Food Diary** for simple steps to get started on monitoring your eating habits.

Portion It

The terms "portion" and "serving size" are often used interchangeably, but they have different meanings in the context of nutrition and food consumption. **A portion is not necessarily a serving size.** Read that last sentence again and make sure you understand that. A serving size is the recommended or standardized measurement of food per day for a 2000-calorie diet. Serving sizes are typically expressed in familiar units such as cups, ounces, grams, or pieces. This quantity is determined by food manufacturers and is often listed on the nutrition facts label on packaged foods to provide you with information about the amount of food considered a single serving. Serving sizes are standardized to allow for easier comparison between various products. However, they may not necessarily represent a recommended or realistic portion for an individual.

A portion is the amount of food or drink that is served as determined by the chef or restaurant, or the amount of food an individual chooses to eat at one time. Portion size is subjective and depends on factors such as personal preferences, hunger, and dietary habits. You may consume portions that are larger or smaller than the standard serving size, impacting the overall caloric and nutrient intake.

It is important for you to be aware of both serving sizes and portions so you can make informed decisions about your individualized dietary intake. Additionally, practicing portion control is often recommended as part of a healthy eating pattern because you can eat too much or too little. **You have control over your portion.** When eating out, if the meal served is too much for you or more than you would like to consume, ask for a to-go box, and take half of your meal home before you clear the entire plate. When you are at home, eat from a plate or bowl, not a package to help manage your portion. Know one pound of body weight equals 3,500 calories, therefore it becomes a balancing act of knowing when too much is too much or when too little is not enough. The benefit of portion control is its flexibility, allowing yourself to indulge in your favorite foods occasionally and stay within your calorie limits. Remember, moderation is key.

Portion control can be challenging, but using visual comparisons with common items can make it easier. Here are some general guidelines for estimating serving sizes:

- **Proteins**
  Meat, poultry, fish: A deck of cards or the palm of your hand (excluding fingers), which is roughly 3 ounces.
  Nut butter: A ping pong ball or a golf ball, which is 2 tablespoons.
  Cheese: Four dice or a pair of thumbs, which is approximately 1.5 ounces.
- **Carbohydrates**
  Cooked pasta or rice: A tennis ball or a fist, which is roughly 1 cup.
  Potato (baked, mashed, etc.): A computer mouse, which is roughly 1 cup.
- **Fruits and Vegetables**
  Fresh fruit: A baseball, which is roughly 1 cup or one medium piece (e.g., an apple or an orange).
  Dried fruit: A golf ball, which is roughly ¼ cup.
  Vegetables: A baseball or a fist, which is roughly 1 cup for raw leafy greens or ½ cup cooked.
- **Dairy**
  Milk or yogurt: A standard 8-ounce cup.
  Cheese (hard): Four dice, or 1.5 ounces.
- **Fats and Oils**
  Butter or margarine: A postage stamp, which is 1 teaspoon.
  Oil: A poker chip, which is 1 tablespoon.
- **Snacks and Sweets**
  Nuts or seeds: A small handful or a golf ball, which is roughly 1 ounce.
  Chocolate: A matchbox or 1 ounce.

Chips or pretzels: A small handful, which is roughly 1 ounce or 15-20 chips.
- **Miscellaneous**
Condiments (like salad dressing): About the size of a shot glass or 2 tablespoons.

Using these visual comparisons can help you gauge serving sizes more accurately without the need for a scale or measuring cups, making it easier to maintain portion control.

Vary It

Consuming a variety of fruits and vegetables is essential for several reasons. Different fruits and vegetables offer a diverse range of nutrients, vitamins, minerals, antioxidants, and other beneficial compounds. Consuming an assortment ensures that you get a broad spectrum of nutrients, helping to meet your body's distinct needs. The antioxidants and phytochemicals found in these foods play a role in protecting the body against oxidative stress and inflammation. They are excellent sources of dietary fiber, which is important for digestive health—helping prevent constipation, promoting regular bowel movements, and contributing to weight management by providing a feeling of fullness. Most fruits and vegetables are low in calories and fat, making them a nutritious choice for those looking to manage their weight or reduce caloric intake, while they are also naturally free of cholesterol. Many fruits and vegetables have high water content, contributing to hydration. Nutrients, such as vitamin C and zinc, play a beneficial role in supporting the immune system. Vitamins A and C contribute to healthy skin by promoting collagen formation, protecting against sun damage, and supporting overall skin health. Many Americans do not get the recommended five or more servings a day of fruit and vegetables, so look for opportunities to add more fruits and veggies to your diet. Choose seasonable vegetables vs. seasoned fries as your side when at a restaurant, add a handful of spinach to your protein shake at home, top your oats with blueberries at breakfast, and dip carrots and peppers in hummus at snack time. Explore the produce aisle and be adventurous by adding a new color of fruits and veggies to your routine. This rainbow of fruits and veggies helps to maintain good health, prevent diseases, and provide the body with the essential nutrients it needs to function optimally. When comparing canned options look for low-sodium vegetables and fruits packed in natural juice and water rather than syrup.

Here are some examples of vegetables representing each color of the rainbow. Challenge yourself to eat one from each color this week:

- **Red**
  Tomatoes
  Red bell peppers
  Radishes
  Red onions
  Beets
- **Orange**
  Carrots
  Sweet potatoes
  Butternut squash
  Orange bell peppers
  Pumpkin
- **Yellow**
  Yellow bell peppers
  Yellow squash
  Yellow tomatoes
  Corn
  Yellow zucchini
- **Green**
  Spinach
  Broccoli
  Kale
  Green beans
  Brussels sprouts
  Asparagus
- **Blue/Purple**
  Eggplant
  Purple cabbage
  Purple potatoes
  Blueberries
  Blackberries
- **White**
  Cauliflower
  White potatoes
  Garlic
  Onions
  Mushrooms

Prep It

If you are one to think that eating healthy, affordable, home-cooked meals on a consistent basis is impossible, you are not alone. Many find it overwhelming to plan a menu, go to the grocery store to pick everything up, and then find the time and energy to prepare it. However, meal planning does become easier the more you do it and can save you time and money in the end, while also putting you in control over what you eat. The key to successful meal planning is to establish a routine or system that works for you.

First, decide how much you are willing to spend and what you want to eat each week. Take the time to write out a menu for each week with a budget. Over a four-week period you now have a month of meals that you can repeat from month to month. Decide what you want to make for breakfasts, lunches, dinners, and snacks. If you have a few go-to meals that you love, then repeat them as needed or wanted. There is no need to search for new recipes every week when you have a few favorites that are the perfect fallbacks. Also try to stretch your proteins by cooking once and eating them more than once. Are you a family that likes grilled chicken breasts? Then bulk grill a family pack or two (large packs are frequently on sale) on Sunday and add a sweet potato and steamed broccoli to make your first meal. On Monday, use that chicken again on a bed of leafy greens with extra salad toppings or create a southwestern chicken wrap. On Tuesday, create one more meal with cauliflower fried rice or add to a stir-fry. This allows you to extend the protein using it as a leftover without having to eat the exact same meal three times leading to boredom. In **Figure 4-1** on the next page, you can see an example of a simple monthly meal planner. Turn to **Worksheet E: Monthly Meal Planners** for a blank template you can use.

Prepare your grocery lists. Are there items you purchase every week? Keep a list on your phone with items you buy on a regular basis: chicken, apples, eggs, milk, bread, etc. These items are your staples. Break the additional items you need to purchase into categories to make your shopping more effective: fresh, non-perishables, refrigerated and deli, frozen, miscellaneous. To stay on budget, peruse the weekly grocery store flyer or app to help you make your list. When you are shopping, stick to the grocery list and never shop while hungry. You will be less likely to make impulse purchases or grab extra food that ends up going to waste by the end of the week. Also try to speed past the less-healthy food options. If you skip over the ultra-processed food aisles such as cookies and chips, you can miss the temptations that are often difficult to resist. Good luck at the check-out! There is no avoiding the extras they place there to tempt you while you are waiting for the cashier or the next available self-check out to open. This is simply discipline and you might need to bring out your superpowers to avoid buying them.

Utilizing a grocery list organizer and/or grocery shopping checklist streamlines the shopping experience, helping to efficiently plan meals,

FIGURE 4-1: Sample Monthly Meal Planner

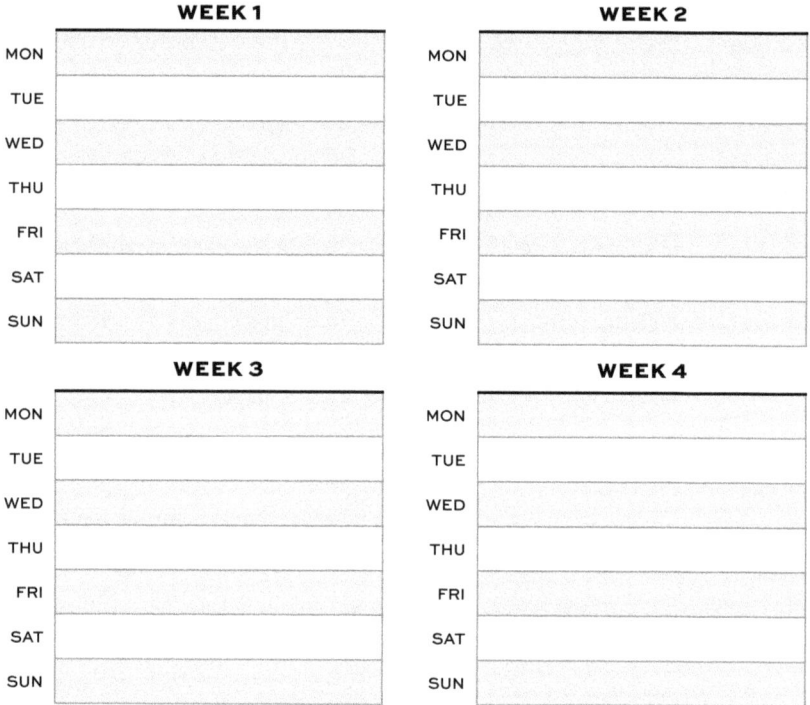

track inventory, and ensure all essential items are purchased. Turn to **Worksheet F: Grocery List Organizer** and **Worksheet G: Grocery Shopping Checklist** to use these tools.

Stock up on items that you can store in your pantry or freezer for quick-need nights. Buying in bulk can also be friendly on the budget so keep your eye out for deals. Some good bulk buying options include beans, frozen veggies, grains, rice, seeds, and nuts. If protein and produce are on sale, buy them and freeze the extras. Consider getting a food saver that vacuum seals. You can buy in bulk at the store, come home and split the bulk portions into smaller portions, vacuum seal, and then freeze until later.

Decide if you are going to need to shop multiple times and if so, what day(s) you can fit it into your schedule. Planning is part of the game. Now you know if you can get to the store yourself, if you need to send someone else, or if you need to have your groceries delivered.

Spend time meal prepping by bulk cooking your protein, washing, and cutting up your veggies, and making snack bags (remember portion control). You might consider creating a weekly "prep" day to get ready for your upcoming meals. It is also a clever idea to double recipes if you want leftovers or can freeze a portion of the meal for the following week. I have learned some people love leftovers while others do not... you know who you are.

If cooking isn't your forte, perhaps you're more of a food system buyer. Many companies and restaurants offer pre-made snacks and meal choices, eliminating the need for time spent on shopping, prepping, and cooking. At the end of the day, you just need to be honest with yourself and discover what system works best for you. No guilt if you did not inherit the Top Chef gene. During particularly busy weeks, I rely on my local small businesses that offer pre-made meals. Grabbing a salad, soup, or protein bowl is sometimes exactly what is needed when I know I will be running short on time. Plan either way, whatever works for you, and execute your plan to successful healthy eating. See **Figure 4-2** on the next page for an example of a weekly meal planner.

Cook It

When choosing healthier cooking methods, you're not only enhancing the flavors and textures of your meals but also promoting your overall well-being. There are various cooking techniques you can consider:

- **Steam:** Steaming involves cooking food over boiling water, which helps retain vitamins and minerals. Invest in a steamer basket or use a simple pot with a lid. Steam broccoli, carrots, cauliflower, or green beans until tender-crisp for a vibrant side dish. Steam delicate fish fillets or shrimp with herbs and a splash of citrus for a light and healthy meal. Enjoy fluffy and perfectly cooked quinoa or brown rice by steaming them in a pot with water or broth.
- **Sauté with Healthy Oils:** Sautéing is a cooking technique that involves cooking food quickly in a small amount of oil or fat over relatively high heat. By choosing heart-healthy oils like olive oil, avocado oil, or coconut oil, you not only enhance the flavor and

FIGURE 4-2: Sample Weekly Meal Planner

	BREAKFAST	LUNCH	DINNER
MON			
TUE			
WED			
THU			
FRI			
SAT			
SUN			

THIS WEEK'S SNACKS

SHOPPING LIST

FAMILY SUGGESTIONS

texture of your dishes, but you also support your cardiovascular health by providing beneficial fats and antioxidants. Sauté leafy greens such as spinach or kale with garlic and a drizzle of olive oil for a nutritious side dish. Cook diced onions, bell peppers, and lean ground turkey or tempeh for a flavorful taco filling. Sauté shrimp or scallops with cherry tomatoes, fresh herbs, and a splash of white wine for an elegant seafood dish.

- **Grill or Broil:** Grilling and broiling are excellent methods for cooking meats, fish, and vegetables without adding extra fats. Marinate proteins with healthy herbs, spices, and citrus juices to enhance flavor. Grill colorful bell peppers, zucchini, eggplant, and mushrooms for a flavorful vegetable medley. Fire up the grill for lean cuts of meat like chicken breasts, turkey burgers, or pork tenderloin. Get creative with grilled fruit skewers, such as pineapple, peaches, and strawberries, for a naturally sweet dessert or snack.

- **Bake or Roast Foods:** Baking and roasting allow foods to cook in their juices, preserving flavors and nutrients. Use parchment paper or a light coating of oil to prevent sticking. Try baking sweet potatoes, butternut squash, or Brussels sprouts for a caramelized, crispy texture. Bake chicken breasts or fish fillets with herbs and spices for a flavorful and tender main dish. Roast root vegetables such as carrots, parsnips, and beets with a sprinkle of herbs for a hearty side dish.
- **Stir-Fry:** Stir-frying involves cooking food quickly over high heat with minimal oil. Use a non-stick pan or wok and load up on colorful veggies, lean proteins, and flavorful sauces. Stir-fry bell peppers, snap peas, broccoli, and tofu or chicken in a wok with a splash of soy sauce and ginger. Create a delicious and nutritious stir-fry using brown rice or quinoa as a base, loaded with your favorite veggies and lean protein. Explore different stir-fry sauces made with ingredients like low-sodium soy sauce, garlic, honey, and sesame oil for a burst of flavor.
- **Poach:** Poaching involves gently simmering food in water or broth. This method works well for fish, chicken, eggs, and fruits. It retains moisture and prevents the need for added fats. Poach chicken breasts in broth with aromatics like garlic, ginger, and lemongrass for a flavorful and tender result. Poach eggs for a nutritious breakfast or brunch option, served over whole grain toast or a bed of sautéed greens. Poach fruits like pears or apples in a spiced syrup for a comforting and healthy dessert.

Hurdle It

Even the best thought-out systems need a contingency plan, and making dinner is no exception. Be prepared for the unexpected situations that may arise while cooking. Whether it is a power outage, getting stuck in traffic, the gas tank that ran out for the grill, forgetting to turn on the crockpot, that one ingredient you forgot at the store, the late-night meeting or practice that ran late, burnt or overcooked food, or kitchen equipment failure—life happens so be ready with a Plan B. Here are some tips for what I like to call "disaster recovery":

- Keep non-perishable foods that require minimal or no cooking, on hand (canned goods, ready-to-eat items, steam veggie packages, frozen meals).
- Have alternative cooking methods available (a gas stove, an air fryer, a portable grill, an extra tank for the grill).
- Have a list of quick and simple recipes that use common ingredients.
- Plan and prep ingredients in advance.
- Know what local restaurants serve quick, healthy, grab-and-go options.

Finally, be ready to make the *best bad choice*. The phrase "make the best bad choice" came from a client of mine who once called me in a panic. She was at work in back-to-back all-day meetings, and she said, "I forgot to pack my snacks, I'm standing in front of a vending machine, help me make my best bad choice!" After we had a good laugh, I asked her to tell me her options—fruit snacks, chocolate donuts, an assortment of chips, gum, hard candies, and candy bars, one of which was a Snickers. We chose Snickers. Was it the best bad choice? Maybe. Maybe not. Let's face it, sometimes we just need something to get us by at the time and truly improvise. If you are at home and frozen pizza is the best bad choice, try to throw a fruit or vegetable with it and do not let one meal that did not go as planned sabotage the rest of your week.

Organize It

Create a healthy eating environment by organizing your kitchen and dining room. Clear the clutter from the countertops to create a clean and open workspace. Purge items you do not use or need. Remove any ultra-processed or junk foods from your pantry, fridge, and freezer. This includes sugary snacks, chips, cookies, candy, soda, and ultra-processed meats. Declutter the condiments in your fridge and the expired spices in your pantry, preparing the space for updated and fresh ingredients. Arrange items by categories such as baking supplies, pots and pans, utensils, spices, etc. Install shelves, cabinets, and hooks for storing extra dishes, glasses, and cookware. Purchase baskets, jars, or containers to use in the refrigerator and pantry for healthy snacks and easy-to-go grabs for lunches. Choose clear containers and jars to see contents easily and keep track of how much you have at any given time. Label the containers and jars to easily identify contents, especially for items like flour, sugar, and spices. Keep healthy snacks visible in a stylish bowl on the counter or in the center of your kitchen table and put the less healthy food out of sight. Create a command center by designating a space for important items. This can include a central area for mail, keys, chargers, and other daily essentials; and a bulletin board or calendar to keep track of grocery lists, schedules, and important reminders. Create an inviting kitchen table, and dining room free of distractions, so you can sit and enjoy a meal. This might mean you have to find a new workstation for that at-home office or a better place for the sports bag and extra shoes that come into the house. Schedule regular cleanouts to get rid of expired items and declutter. As your needs change, be flexible with your organization and adjust accordingly. Remember, the key to an organized kitchen is to create a system that works for you and to maintain it regularly. Customizing your organization strategy based on your cooking habits and lifestyle will help keep your kitchen functional and enjoyable to use.

Savor It

How many times do you find yourself rushing through your meals, eating on the go, scrolling your phone at the table, watching the game, or binging a show on the couch? Slow down! Savoring your food involves fully engaging your senses and appreciating the flavors, textures, and aromas of what you are eating. Start by being present while you eat. Focus on the moment and pay attention to your meal as you eliminate distractions. Turn off the TV, put away your phone, stop working at your desk, and sit at the table. Take a moment to smell your food. The sense of smell is intricately linked to taste, and it can enhance your overall dining experience. Use your eyes to appreciate the colors, shapes, and presentation of your food. Feel the textures of food in your mouth. Notice if it is hot, cold, hard, soft, smooth, or crunchy. Pay attention to the different flavors. Try to identify specific tastes, such as sweet, salty, bitter, and sour. Learn to slow down. Chew your food thoroughly. This not only allows you to savor the flavors but also aids in digestion. Listen to your body's hunger and fullness cues and realize it takes approximately twenty minutes for your brain to signal that your stomach is full. Do not start putting the next bite onto your fork until you have finished chewing and swallowing your previous bite. Drink water in between bites and place your fork down while you chew. Appreciate how healthy food will fuel your body to perform optimally, and taste layers of flavors as you savor each bite. Experiment with new dishes, fresh herbs, different spices, various cooking techniques. Discover flavors from diverse cultures, pair your meal with a beverage that complements its flavors. Share the meal with friends and family to enhance the experience and create a positive association with food.

Hydrate It

Approximately 60 percent of an adult human body is composed of water. Therefore, staying hydrated is important for the proper functioning of the body. Water plays a vital role in various physiological processes. Starting at the cellular level, water helps transport nutrients into the cells and removes waste products from them. Proper cell function leads to optimized activity of the tissues, organs, and organ systems. When your body is properly hydrated, it efficiently regulates your body temperature through the process of sweating. Too little water leads to dehydration and the possibility of overheating or heat-related illnesses. Being dehydrated can also impair cognitive function, including your attention span, memory, and concentration. Water is a major component of synovial fluid, which lubricates joints. Proper joint lubrication is essential for smooth movement and to prevent discomfort or pain associated with friction between joints.

When it comes to the digestion of food and the absorption of nutrients, water helps break down food particles and facilitates the movement of nutrients across the digestive tract and into the bloodstream. Blood is composed of approximately 50–55 percent water, and adequate hydration helps maintain proper blood volume and viscosity. This, in turn, supports the efficient transport of oxygen and nutrients to cells and the removal of waste products in the blood. Hydration helps ensure the proper balance of electrolytes in the body which includes minerals such as sodium, potassium, and chloride. These electrolytes carry an electric charge and play a crucial role in maintaining fluid balance, nerve function, and muscle contractions. Proper hydration supports the function of the kidneys in filtering and excreting waste materials primarily through urine. Hydration also affects how our skin feels and looks. Well-hydrated skin is more elastic and less prone to dryness and irritation, promoting a healthy, vibrant appearance. Drinking water before and during meals may affect how full you feel since being dehydrated is often mistaken for hunger. It is important to note that individual water needs vary based on factors such as age, sex, activity level, and climate. As a general rule drink half your weight in water (in ounces) while listening to your body's signals.

The biggest piece of advice I can offer when drinking water is to find what works for you. Do you drink more water with a straw or straight out of a cup, when it is ice cold or room temperature, plain or with a hint of natural fruit juice, from a glass or plastic water bottle, always carrying it around or leaving multiple bottles around the house and workstations, filtered or straight out of the tap? I encourage you to find what gets you excited about drinking water and start tracking your consumption. Set reminders and use alarms or hydration tracking apps to remind you to drink water throughout the day.

Hydration tips for getting in 8 glasses of water a day:

- Drink a glass of water when you wake up to activate your organs.
- Drink a glass of water before you eat breakfast, lunch, and dinner to help with digestion.
- Drink a glass of water before you take a shower.
- Drink a glass of water during and after activity to replenish what you have lost through perspiration.
- Drink a glass of water before your bedtime snack.

Jazz up your hydration with some simple twists:

- **Citrus Infusions:** Squeeze fresh lemon, lime, or orange slices into your water for a zesty burst of flavor. For an extra kick, add a few sprigs of fresh mint or a slice of cucumber. It's like spa water, right at home!
- **Berry Bliss:** Drop a handful of berries—like strawberries, blueberries, raspberries, or blackberries—into your water for a sweet and tangy upgrade. The berries not only add flavor but also infuse your water with antioxidants.
- **Herbal Elegance:** Fresh herbs can take your hydration game to the next level. Add sprigs of rosemary, basil, thyme, or lavender to your water for a subtle, aromatic twist.
- **Tropical Paradise:** Transport yourself to a sunny beach with a splash of tropical fruits. Pineapple chunks, mango slices, or a hint of coconut water can transform your water into a vacation in a glass.
- **Cucumber Cooler:** Cool as a cucumber—literally! Thinly slice cucumber and let it infuse in your water for a crisp and refreshing drink. Add a squeeze of lime for a tangy twist.
- **Spice It Up:** Feeling adventurous? Try adding a dash of spice to your water. A pinch of cayenne pepper, ginger slices, or a cinnamon stick can add a unique flavor kick and boost your metabolism.
- **Fizz and Fun:** If you love the effervescence of soda but want a healthier option, try sparkling water. Add a splash of 100-percent fruit juice, a twist of lime, or some muddled berries for a bubbly, guilt-free treat.
- **DIY Tea Infusions:** Brew a batch of your favorite herbal tea, let it cool, and then chill it in the fridge. Add this tea concentrate to your water for a refreshing and hydrating beverage with added health benefits.

Get creative and mix different fruits, herbs, and spices to create your signature water concoction. The possibilities are endless, so have fun experimenting! Remember, staying hydrated doesn't have to be boring.

With a little creativity and some fresh ingredients, you can transform plain water into a delicious and revitalizing drink.

SWAP It

Learn to SWAP out healthier options. **SWAP** = **S**witch **W**ith **A P**ositive. The goal is to make simple changes to your diet and replace less healthy foods with more nutritious foods. See **Figure 4-3** below for some suggested SWAP options.

FIGURE 4-3: Suggested SWAP options

REPLACE THIS	WITH THIS
Processed snacks	Fresh fruit or homemade trail mix
White bread	Whole grain or sprouted bread
Regular pasta	Zucchini noodles or lentil pasta
Soda	Seltzer water or green tea
Fruit juice	Whole fruit or fruit-infused water
Artificial sweeteners	Honey or stevia
Mayo	Avocado
Ketchup	Salsa
Milk chocolate	Dark chocolate
Sugary cereal	Oatmeal
Chips	Sliced veggies or homemade veggie chips
Butter	Olive or avocado oil
Hamburger	Fish
Bagel	English muffin
Flavored yogurt	Plain yogurt with berries
Sour cream	Greek yogurt
White rice	Quinoa or cauliflower rice
Tortillas	Lettuce wraps
Sugar	Stevia or honey
Ice cream	Frozen yogurt or banana ice cream
Cream-based soups	Broth-based soups
Croutons	Nuts or seeds
Mashed potatoes	Mashed cauliflower

Control It

Maintaining healthy eating habits can be challenging when your routine is disrupted by dining out, social events, family gatherings, or holiday celebrations. During these unstructured times, it's essential to have strategies in place to direct your food and beverage intake without feeling deprived or out of place. By being mindful and prepared, you can enjoy these occasions while staying aligned with your health and wellness goals. Here are a few ideas for how you can effectively manage your choices and ensure a balanced approach to eating and drinking during these special events:

AT A RESTAURANT
- **Plan ahead:** Review the menu online before going and choose healthier options.
- **Start with a salad or soup:** Opt for a salad with dressing on the side or a broth-based soup to fill up on low-calorie options.
- **Choose grilled, baked, or steamed:** Avoid fried foods and remember the healthy cooking options we talked about earlier in this chapter.
- **Ask for modifications:** Request for dressings and sauces on the side and ask if the dish can be prepared with less oil or butter (sometimes you can ask for a "heart healthy" option).
- **Portion control:** Consider sharing a dish or asking for a half-portion. You can also ask for a to-go box at the start and portion out half of your meal to take home.
- **Skip the bread basket and/or chips and salsa:** If it's a temptation, kindly ask the server to remove it or not bring it to the table.
- **Choose water or unsweetened beverages:** Avoid sugary drinks and opt for water, sparkling water, or unsweetened tea.
- **Limit alcohol:** If you drink, stick to one glass, and opt for wine or light beer instead of sugary cocktails.
- **Mind your sides:** Choose healthier sides like veggies, a side salad, or a baked potato instead of fries or creamy dishes.

- **Dessert strategy:** If you want dessert, consider sharing it or choosing a fruit-based option.

AT FAMILY, SOCIAL, OR HOLIDAY GATHERINGS
- **Eat before you go:** Have a healthy snack or small meal before arriving to avoid overeating.
- **Bring a healthy dish:** Offer to bring a dish you know is healthy to ensure there's at least one good option available.
- **Survey the spread:** Look at all the food options before filling your plate to make mindful choices.
- **Use a smaller plate:** Control portion sizes by tricking your eye with a smaller plate.
- **Fill half your plate with vegetables:** Load up on non-starchy veggies first to help fill you up.
- **Be selective with treats:** Choose your favorite holiday treats and savor them but avoid mindlessly snacking on everything.
- **Drink plenty of water:** Stay hydrated, which can help prevent overeating.
- **Limit high-calorie drinks:** Be mindful in beverages like eggnog, soda, and alcoholic drinks.
- **Focus on socializing:** Spend more time engaging with family and friends rather than hovering around the food.

Build It

You are the architect of your nutrition. You get to plan, design, and construct what you eat and drink. Focus on high-quality, nutrient-dense foods while limiting or eliminating energy-dense foods and realize that portion control does matter because *you cannot outrun your fork*. Let's break this down into macronutrients and micronutrients.

Macronutrients describe the three main nutrients we receive from food that the human body requires in relatively large amounts to function properly, thus the macro part of that word. They are proteins, carbohydrates, and fats. *Micronutrients* describe the nutrients we need in smaller amounts, which are needed for normal growth and development. These are our minerals and vitamins.

PROTEIN

Proteins are an essential macronutrient that play an important role in promoting various functions within the human body. Composed of twenty different amino acids, they are involved in numerous processes essential for life. Structural proteins maintain and protect the structural integrity and proper function of the cells, tissues, and organs. Examples include collagen in skin and keratin in hair. Many proteins act as enzymes, facilitating and catalyzing chemical reactions in the body. They are essential for bodily functions such as your digestion, energy production, and DNA replication. Some proteins function as hormones, acting as signaling molecules that regulate physiological processes and maintain homeostasis. For example, insulin regulates blood sugar levels, and growth hormones influence growth and development of our bodies. Antibodies are specialized proteins that recognize and neutralize foreign substances (antigens) like pathogens, helping the immune system defend against infections. Some proteins transport molecules such as oxygen (hemoglobin), ions, and nutrients across cell membranes or through the bloodstream. Muscle function is affected by protein because muscle tissue is rich in proteins, particularly contractile proteins like actin and myosin. These proteins enable muscle contraction, allowing for movement and physical activity. While carbohydrates and fats are the primary energy sources, the body can use protein for energy when needed. However, this is not the preferred source, and it usually occurs under certain conditions like prolonged fasting or intense exercise.

It is important to note that the functions of proteins are diverse and interconnected, and critical for the overall health and proper functioning of the body. A balanced and varied diet is integral in providing the necessary amino acids for the syntheses of these proteins to support these essential functions.

The Food and Drug Administration's (FDA) Dietary Guidelines for Americans recommends a daily allowance of protein in your diet at 10–35 percent of your total calories.[9] As a general guideline, sedentary adults need 0.8 grams of protein per kilogram of body weight, while active individuals need 1.2-2.2 grams of protein per kilogram of body weight. Athletes, pregnant and breastfeeding women, and those recovering from illness or surgery may require higher amounts of protein. Additionally, dietary preferences such as vegetarian or vegan diets may require careful planning to ensure adequate protein intake from plant-based sources. The most efficient way to achieve the proper amount of dietary protein is to include protein in every meal and every snack throughout your day.

Great sources of protein consist of grilled chicken, turkey breast, ground turkey, game meats like venison, salmon, halibut, cod, shellfish, lean red meat, lamb, eggs, pork tenderloin, Greek yogurt, cottage cheese, chickpeas, lentils, tofu, edamame, quinoa, kidney beans, hemp seeds, pumpkin seeds, black beans, sunflower seeds, almonds, flax seeds, cashews, chia seeds, and plant-based protein powder consisting of pea protein, rice protein, and hemp protein. It is important to note that while animal-based sources of protein usually provide all essential amino acids, some plant-based sources may lack one or more amino acids.

Whether you're planning breakfast, lunch, dinner, or snacks, focusing on protein-rich foods can help you meet your nutritional goals. Here are some excellent examples of high-protein options for each meal that are both delicious and nutritious:

Breakfast
- Greek yogurt topped with nuts and berries
- Scrambled eggs with spinach and feta cheese
- Protein smoothie with protein powder, your choice of milk or water, and a handful of spinach
- Overnight oats made with chia seeds, almond butter, and a sprinkle of hemp hearts

Lunch
- Grilled chicken or tofu on a bed of mixed greens with avocado and vinaigrette

---

[9] Dietary Guidelines for Americans. 2020-2025. Make Every Bite Count with the Dietary Guidelines. 9th ed. Dietaryguidelines.gov. US Department of Health and Human Services and U.S. Department of Agriculture. (2020). Dietary Guidelines for Americans. Retrieved from https://www.dietaryguidelines.gov/sites/default/files/2020-12/Dietary_Guidelines_for_Amerians_2020-2025.pdf

- Quinoa salad with chickpeas, cucumbers, cherry tomatoes, and a lemon-tahini dressing
- Turkey and cheese roll-ups with lettuce, tomato, and mustard in a whole grain wrap
- Lentil soup with a side of whole grain bread and a dollop of Greek yogurt

Dinner
- Baked salmon with roasted asparagus and quinoa
- Tofu stir-fry with broccoli, bell peppers, and a ginger-soy sauce
- Lean beef or turkey meatballs served over zucchini noodles with marinara sauce
- Chickpea and vegetable curry served with brown rice

Snacks
- A small handful of almonds or walnuts
- Cottage cheese with a drizzle of honey and a sprinkle of cinnamon
- Sliced hard-boiled eggs with a pinch of sea salt
- Protein shake made with your choice of protein powder and milk or water
- Almond butter or hummus with carrot sticks or apple slices
- Roasted chickpeas seasoned with your favorite spices
- Beef or turkey jerky for a savory, on-the-go option

CARBOHYDRATES

Carbohydrates (aka carbs) are composed of carbon, hydrogen, and oxygen atoms. They are the body's primary and preferred source of energy. When consumed, they are broken down into glucose ($C_6H_{12}O_6$), also known as blood sugar, which is then used by cells for fuel. Adequate carbohydrate intake spares proteins from being used as an energy source. When the body lacks carbohydrates, it may resort to breaking down proteins for energy. This can be detrimental to maintaining muscle mass if you are not consuming enough protein. If you have excess glucose, it is stored in the liver and muscles in the form of glycogen. This glycogen serves as a reserve that can be quickly converted back into glucose when the body needs an extra energy boost, such as during exercize or fasting. Glucose is also the preferred energy source for the brain. Certain carbs, such as dietary fiber, promote digestive health by adding bulk to stool, aiding in bowel movements, and supporting the growth of beneficial gut bacteria. Fiber also helps regulate blood glucose levels as it slows the absorption of glucose and improves insulin sensitivity, contributing to stable blood sugar levels. Carbs also contribute to the taste and palatability of many foods. They are often a key component in the flavor profile of various foods, making them more enjoyable and satisfying.

It is important to note that not all carbohydrates are the same. Carbs are broadly classified into three main types based on their structure: monosaccharides, disaccharides, and polysaccharides.

- **Monosaccharides** are the simplest form of carbs, consisting of a single sugar molecule. Examples include glucose, fructose, and galactose. These guys are the building blocks of more complex carbs.
- **Disaccharides** are formed by the combination of two monosaccharide molecules. For example: glucose + fructose = sucrose; glucose + galactose = lactose; and glucose + glucose = maltose. These disaccharides are broken down into monosaccharides during digestion.
- **Polysaccharides** are large, complex molecules composed of multiple monosaccharide units. Here we have starch which is found in plants and used as a storage form of glucose. Cellulose is a structural polysaccharide found in the cell walls of plants that provide rigidity and support. Also, chitin, which is found in the exoskeletons of arthropods and in the cell walls of fungi, provides structural support.

The Dietary Guidelines for Americans recommend that carbohydrates make up 45–65 percent of total daily calories.[9] So if you get 2,000 calories a day, between 900 and 1,300 calories should be from carbohydrates. That translates to between 225 and 325 grams of carbs a day. Recommendations from the American Heart Association (AHA) advises consumption of added sugars be only 5 percent of daily calories.[10] For adult women, this would be fewer than 100 calories (about 25 grams or 6 teaspoons) per day, and for adult men, fewer than 150 calories (about 37.5 grams or 9 teaspoons) per day. The Institute of Medicine (IOM) has also set adequate intakes for dietary fiber at 25 grams for women and 38 grams for men.[11] This recommendation for dietary fiber is based on the intake levels known to prevent heart disease. The Food and Nutrition Board of IOM has set the Recommended Dietary Allowance (RDA) of carbohydrates for children and adults at 130 grams per day.[9] This is often considered a minimum requirement the brain requires to function properly. Individuals who engage in high levels of physical activity, especially endurance athletes, may require a higher percentage of calories from carbohydrates to support their energy needs. It is important to note that people have different responses to macronutrient ratios, and there is no one-size-fits-all recommendation. Some individuals may feel better with a higher or lower carbohydrate intake.

Additionally, the type of carbohydrate matters. Choose whole, unprocessed foods like brown rice, quinoa, oats, barley, and whole wheat. Whole grains are considered healthier than refined grains because they contain more nutrients and fiber. In contrast, refined grains have had the bran and germ removed, leaving only the endosperm. This process removes some of the nutrients and fiber present in the whole grain. When people talk about "whole carbs" in dietary context, they are often referring to carbohydrates obtained from whole, un-processed sources like fruits, vegetables, and whole grains, as opposed to refined or ultra-processed carbs. These whole carbs provide a more complete and nutritious package, including fiber, vitamins, and minerals.

---

[10] Johnson, R. K., L. J. Appel, M. Brands, B. V. Howard, M. Lefevre, R. H. Lustig, F. Sacks, L. M. Steffen, J. Wylie-Rosett, and on behalf of the American Heart Association Nutrition Committee of the Council on Nutrition, Physical Activity, and Metabolism and the Council on Epidemiology and Prevention. 2010. Dietary sugars intake and cardiovascular health: A scientific statement from the American Heart Association. Circulation 120:1011–1020. [PubMed]

[11] Trumbo P, Schlicker S, Yates AA, Poos M; Food and Nutrition Board of the Institute of Medicine, The National Academies. Dietary reference intakes for energy, carbohydrate, fiber, fat, fatty acids, cholesterol, protein, and amino acids. J Am Diet Assoc. 2002 Nov;102(11):1621-30. doi: 10.1016/s0002-8223(02)90346-9. Erratum in: J Am Diet Assoc. 2003 May;103(5):563. PMID: 12449285.

When planning breakfast, lunch, dinner, or snacks, incorporating nutritious, carbohydrate-rich foods can help keep you energized and satisfied. Here are some excellent examples of high-carbohydrate options for each meal that are both delicious and nutritious:

Breakfast
- Oatmeal with mixed berries (blueberries, strawberries), a handful of nuts (almonds, walnuts), and a drizzle of honey or maple syrup
- Whole grain toast topped with a mashed avocado, a sprinkle of salt and pepper, cherry tomatoes, and a poached egg
- Smoothie bowl made with banana, spinach, Greek yogurt, chia seeds, granola, and a variety of fruits like mango and kiwi
- Veggie omelet with eggs or egg whites, fresh spinach, cherry tomatoes, chopped onions and optional cheese

Lunch
- Quinoa salad made with cooked quinoa, mixed greens, cherry tomatoes, cucumber, chickpeas, feta cheese, olive oil, and lemon juice dressing
- Whole wheat tortilla, grilled chicken or tofu, hummus, spinach, bell peppers, and shredded carrots rolled into a wrap
- Lentil soup with lentils, diced tomatoes, carrots, celery, onions, vegetable broth, and spices like cumin and turmeric
- Tuna salad with mixed greens salad and whole grain crackers

Dinner
- Brown rice stir-fry made with brown rice, mixed vegetables (broccoli, bell peppers, snap peas), tofu or shrimp, soy sauce, and sesame seeds
- Whole grain tortillas, roasted sweet potatoes, black beans, avocado, salsa, and a sprinkle of cheese for taco night
- Spaghetti squash, marinara sauce, ground turkey or meatballs (optional), and a sprinkle of parmesan cheese
- Baked salmon with quinoa and roasted vegetables

Snacks
- Apple slices and your choice of nut butter (peanut, almond)
- Plain Greek yogurt, a handful of granola, and a drizzle of honey
- Carrot sticks, celery sticks, cucumber slices, and hummus
- Chia pudding made with chia seeds, almond milk, a touch of vanilla extract, and topped with fresh berries
- Mixed nuts and seeds (almonds, walnuts, pumpkin seeds, and sunflower seeds)
- Cottage cheese with pineapple chunks
- Whole grain crackers with mashed avocado

Getting to Know the Glycemic Index

This is an appropriate time to discuss the glycemic index (GI). The glycemic index is a value used to measure how quickly a carbohydrate-containing food raises blood glucose levels. Foods are classified as low, medium, or high glycemic foods and ranked on a scale from 0 to 100. Foods with a low GI are those that are digested and absorbed slowly, leading to a slower and more gradual rise in blood sugar levels. These foods are often recommended for people with diabetes or those looking to manage their blood sugar levels. Examples of low-GI foods include most vegetables, legumes, whole grains, and certain fruits. Foods with a high GI are rapidly digested and cause a quick and significant increase in blood sugar levels. These foods are often best consumed in moderation, especially for individuals with diabetes. High-GI foods are high in refined carbs and sugar, and include sugary snacks, white bread, and certain cereals. Besides the quantity and type of carb it contains, other factors that affect the GI of a food include the ripeness, cooking method, type of sugar it contains, and the amount of processing it has undergone.[12]

Choosing foods with a lower glycemic index can be beneficial for managing sugar levels, promoting satiety, and supporting overall health. However, it is essential to consider the overall diet and the individual health goals as the glycemic index is just one factor among many in a healthy eating plan.

GI Levels
Low GI (55 or less): Examples include apples, berries, oranges, lemons, limes, grapefruit, broccoli, cauliflower, carrots, spinach, tomatoes, quinoa, barley, buckwheat, oats, lentils, black beans, chickpeas, kidney beans. **Medium GI (56–69):** Examples include some fruits, whole wheat products, and basmati rice. **High GI (70 or more):** Examples include white bread, bagels, white rice, jasmine rice, instant oats, breakfast cereals, french fries, cookies, donuts, cakes, croissants, muffins, chocolate, crackers, chips, pretzels, soda, fruit juice, sports drinks.

Keep in mind that the glycemic index is different from the glycemic load (GL). The glycemic load considers both the *quality* and *quantity* of carbs in a serving of food and provides a more comprehensive picture of its impact on blood sugar. It is calculated by multiplying the GI of a food by the amount of carbs in a serving and then dividing it by 100.

The formula for calculating glycemic load:

$$\text{Glycemic Load} = \frac{\text{Glycemic Index} \times \text{Carb Content Per Serving (g)}}{100}$$

GL Levels
Low GL (0-10): Foods with a low GL have a smaller impact on blood sugar levels. Examples include most fruits and vegetables. **Medium GL (11–19):** Foods with a moderate GL have a moderate impact on blood sugar levels. Examples include whole grains and some fruits. **High GL (20 and above):** Foods with a high GL can cause a rapid and large increase in blood sugar levels. Examples include sugary foods and processed grains.

Following a low glycemic diet may offer several health benefits including improved blood sugar regulation, increased weight loss, and a reduction in liver fat and liver enzyme levels in people with non-alcoholic fatty liver disease.[13]

FATS

Fats are concentrated sources of energy that play important roles in structural and metabolic functions, including energy storage, waterproofing, and thermal insulation. This macronutrient provides more than twice the energy per gram, compared to carbohydrates and proteins—there are nine calories in every gram of fat and only four calories in every gram of protein and carb (refer to **Figure 4-4**). Fats are a key component of cell membranes. Phospholipids, a type of fat, help form the structural bases of cell membranes, influencing their flexibility and permeability. This is vital for proper cell functioning and signaling. Certain vitamins, such as A, D, E, and K, are fat soluble, meaning they are absorbed better in the presence of fats. Fats help transport these vitamins through the bloodstream and facilitate their absorption in the digestive system. Adipose tissue, which is a type of connective tissue composed mainly of fat cells, acts as an insulating layer under the skin, helping to regulate body temperature by reducing heat loss. It also cushions and protects organs from physical impact. Fats are precursors to produce various hormones. For example, cholesterol, a type of lipid, is a precursor for steroid hormones such as estrogen and testosterone, which play critical roles in reproduction and other physiological processes. The brain contains a significant amount of fat, and certain fats, particularly omega-3 fatty acids, are crucial for proper brain development and function. Fats also contribute to the sensation of satiety, helping you feel full and satisfied after a meal, while enhancing the taste and palatability of food, making meals more enjoyable.

---

[12] Page 73. Front Nutr. 2022; 9: 1025993. Published online 2022 Nov 10. doi: 10.3389/fnut.2022.1025993. PMCID: PMC9684673. PMID: 36438742. Culinary strategies to manage glycemic response in people with type 2 diabetes: A narrative review. Serafin Murillo, 1 , 2 , 3 Ariadna Mallol, 1 Alba Adot, 1Fabiola Juárez, 1 Alba Coll, 1 Isabella Gastaldo, 2and Elena Roura.

[13] Parker A, Kim Y. The Effect of Low Glycemic Index and Glycemic Load Diets on Hepatic Fat Mass, Insulin Resistance, and Blood Lipid Panels in Individuals with Nonalcoholic Fatty Liver Disease. Metab Syndr Relat Disord. 2019 Oct;17(8):389-396. doi: 10.1089/met.2019.0038. Epub 2019 Jul 15. PMID: 31305201.

It is important to note that not all fats are created equal, meaning there are healthy and unhealthy fats. Choosing healthy fats and maintaining a balanced intake is essential for optimizing health. Incorporating sources of healthy fat, like avocados, nuts, seeds, and fatty fish, can contribute positively to your overall well-being. Consuming too much saturated and trans fats, commonly found in ultra-processed and fried foods, can be detrimental to your health and increase the risk of various diseases, such as cardiovascular disease.

According to the Dietary Guidelines for Americans, adults should aim for 20–35 percent of their total calories in the form of healthy fats.[9] Less than 10 percent of total daily calories should come from saturated fat. Trans fat intake should be as low as possible or less than 1 percent of your total calories. The majority of fat intake should come from sources of monounsaturated and polyunsaturated fats. The main reason being that saturated fats tend to raise the low-density lipoprotein (LDL) cholesterol levels in your blood. There is evidence that these high levels increase your risk of heart disease and stroke. This means limiting your intake of red meat, dairy products, baked goods, and fried foods. The important thing about unsaturated fats (for example vegetable oils, fish, and nuts) is that these fats have been linked to the improvement of your blood cholesterol levels, therefore decreasing your risk of heart attack and stroke.

The best way to start eating healthier fats is to focus on raw nuts, seeds, flaxseed, olive oil, olives, avocado, coconut oil, and peanut butter. Eat fats rich in omega-3 fatty acids (alpha-linoleic acid which is a fatty acid found in leafy greens and some nuts) at least twice a week, or 2 grams a day making up 0.6–1.2 percent of your daily intake, omega-6 fatty acids (linoleic acid) at 5–10 percent of your daily intake, choose lean meats or trim visible fat from your meat, and limit your ultra-processed foods and commercial baked goods.

Including foods rich in healthy fats in your meals can enhance both flavor and nutritional value. Whether you're preparing breakfast, lunch, dinner, or snacks, focusing on healthy fat options can contribute to overall well-being. Here are some great examples of meals and snacks that highlight the benefits of healthy fats while being delicious and satisfying.

Breakfast
- Avocado toast topped with a sprinkle of sea salt and red pepper flakes
- Chia seed pudding made with almond milk, topped with fresh berries, and slivered almonds
- Smoked salmon and cream cheese on a whole grain bagel or toast
- A smoothie bowl blended with coconut milk, almond butter, and a handful of spinach

Lunch
- A spinach and strawberry salad with sliced almonds, feta cheese, and a drizzle of olive oil
- Tuna salad made with avocado instead of mayo, served on whole grain bread or lettuce wraps
- Quinoa salad with diced avocado, cherry tomatoes, cucumbers, and a lemon-tahini dressing
- Hummus and veggie wrap with avocado, shredded carrots, and mixed greens

Dinner
- Grilled salmon with a side of roasted Brussels sprouts tossed in olive oil
- Stir-fried tofu with broccoli, bell peppers, and cashews in a sesame-ginger sauce
- Stuffed bell peppers filled with quinoa, black beans, diced avocado, and salsa
- Spaghetti squash with a creamy avocado pesto sauce and cherry tomatoes

Snacks
- A small bowl of air-popped popcorn drizzled with melted coconut oil
- Sliced pear or apple with a wedge of brie cheese
- Dark chocolate squares paired with a handful of almonds or macadamia nuts

- A smoothie made with coconut milk, frozen berries, and a scoop of almond butter
- A small handful of pumpkin seeds or sunflower seeds
- A serving of olives paired with whole grain crackers or a piece of cheese
- Homemade guacamole with whole grain tortilla chips or veggie sticks for dipping

Each macronutrient provides a certain number of calories per gram.

FIGURE 4-4: Macronutrient calories

NUTRITION	CALORIES PER GRAM
Protein	4
Carbohydrate	4
Fat	9

MICRONUTRIENTS

Micronutrients are defined as vitamins and minerals needed by the body in relatively small amounts for proper growth, development, and overall health. They perform a variety of physiological processes and with the exception of vitamin D, micronutrients are not produced in the body, and therefore, must be attained from your diet. Here's a quick breakdown of micronutrients:

- **Fat-soluble vitamins:** These include vitamins A, D, E, and K, which are soluble in fat and oils and stored in the body for longer periods.
- **Water-soluble vitamins:** This category contains nine vitamins including all the B-vitamins (Riboflavin, Niacin, Thiamin, B6, Folate, B12, Pantothenic Acid, and Biotin) and vitamin C. Water-soluble vitamins are not stored in the body for extended periods but are excreted in urine, so they need to be consumed regularly.
- **Major minerals:** These are needed by the body in amounts larger than 100 milligrams and include calcium, phosphorus, magnesium, sodium, potassium, chloride, and sulfur.

- **Trace minerals:** Are classified as minerals required in the diet each day in smaller amounts, specifically 100 milligrams or less. These include iron, zinc, copper, manganese, iodine, selenium, chromium, fluoride, molybdenum, and others.

Here are the main roles of micronutrients:

- **Cofactors for enzymes:** Many vitamins and minerals act as cofactors or coenzymes for enzymes, facilitating biochemical reactions in the body. For examples, minerals like magnesium and zinc are essential for the activity of numerous enzymes involved in metabolism.
- **Antioxidant defense:** Certain vitamins (e.g., vitamin C, vitamin E) and minerals (e.g., selenium, zinc) act as antioxidants, helping to neutralize free radicals and reduce oxidative stress, which can damage cells and contribute to aging and disease.
- **Energy production:** Several B vitamins (e.g., thiamine, riboflavin, niacin, pantothenic acid) play critical roles in energy metabolism by aiding in the conversion of carbs, fats, and proteins into energy that the body can use.
- **Bone health:** Minerals such as calcium, phosphorus, magnesium, and vitamin D are essential for maintaining strong bones and teeth. They contribute to bone formation, density, and remodeling processes throughout life.
- **Immune function:** Vitamins A, C, D, E, and minerals like zinc and selenium support immune function by promoting the production and activity or immune cells, enhancing the body's ability to fight infections and maintain immune balance.
- **Blood clotting and wound healing:** Vitamin K is crucial for blood clotting, ensuring that wounds heal properly and preventing excessive bleeding.
- **Nervous system function:** Vitamins such as B6, B12, and folate play roles in nerve function, neurotransmitter synthesis, and the maintenance of myelin sheaths that insulate nerves.
- **Vision:** Vitamin A is essential for vision, particularly in low-light

conditions, and helps maintain the health of the retina and other structures of the eye.
- **Metabolic regulation:** Micronutrients help regulate various metabolic pathways, hormone synthesis, and cellular processes essential for growth, development, and maintenance of tissues.

I would like to believe we are all eating the rainbow of fruits and vegetables every day, while also getting the perfect amount and combination of proteins, carbs, and fats to keep our bodies functioning at an optimal level. But the reality is we consume too many ultra-processed foods that have been grown in less-than-perfect environmental conditions and depleted of their nutrients. Micronutrient deficiencies are linked to health conditions, decreased energy levels, and reduction in mental clarity. This then cascades into a decrease in our work productivity and an increased risk of additional diseases. For this reason, adding dietary supplements to your daily regimen may be beneficial, but it is advised to consult with a healthcare professional before taking supplements, as excessive intake can have adverse effects. Also know that price is not necessarily equivalent to quality when it comes to supplements. Check for a product with the United States Pharmacopeia (USP) seal to ensure quality manufacturing integrity. The USP is a comprehensive collection of drug information published by the United States Pharmacopeial Convention, a non-profit organization. The USP sets standards for the equality, purity, strength, and consistency of drugs, food ingredients, and dietary supplements. The USP seal is given to products that have been evaluated by the USP to determine the product has "truth in labeling" meaning, the supplement contains what it claims to contain.

GUT HEALTH

Gut health is absolutely a topic that should be at the top of your priority list. The best way to get a healthy gut is by eating a whole-foods diet high in prebiotic (fiber) and probiotic foods. Adding a probiotic to your daily regimen may offer various health benefits, such as supporting digestive health, enhancing the immune system, and potentially helping with conditions like irritable bowel syndrome (IBS) and certain allergic disorders. Probiotics are live microorganisms that provide health benefits when consumed in adequate amounts. These microorganisms are often referred to as "good" or "friendly" bacteria because they can contribute to the balance of the microbial community in your digestive system. The human gastrointestinal tract naturally contains a diverse community of bacteria that play important roles in digestion, nutrient absorption, and overall gut health. These probiotics can be found in fermented foods like yogurt, kefir, sauerkraut, kimchi, and in some dietary supplements. Adding a prebiotic with your probiotic will help to provide a favorable environment for the growth and activity of beneficial bacteria in your gut. Prebiotics are food for probiotics. Common sources of prebiotics include inulin and fructooligosaccharides (FOS) found in foods such as onions, garlic, leeks, bananas, asparagus, and chicory root; galactooligosaccharides (GOT) are found in legumes, certain vegetables, and some grains; and dietary fibers such as soluble fibers are found in oats, barley, and fruits.

INFLAMMATION

Eat with inflammation in mind. Sometimes the foods you love do not love you back. Everyone has different inflammatory triggers, which means there is not a one-size fits all anti-inflammatory protocol. An anti-inflammatory diet is not actually a diet, but rather an overall way of eating. Even if you don't have a chronic condition, certain foods you're sensitive to could raise your inflammation levels. The foods you do and do not eat can prevent inflammation and help soothe your inflammatory responses. Try scaling back on ultra-processed food. If it comes in a bag or a box with a list of ingredients, then pass on it. Examples include baked goods, candy, potato chips, processed deli meat, processed cheese, sugary drinks, fried food, and alcohol. Now focus on whole foods. Remember those one-ingredient foods I was talking about at the beginning of this chapter? Fruits, veggies, eggs, fish, legumes, nuts, seeds, meat, and seafood. Think Mediterranean Diet, which is a diet focused on these whole foods. If needed, you can also try an elimination period where you remove all potential trigger foods for one to two months to help you figure out how the foods you are eating are affecting you. During this time, check to see if you experience clearer skin, decreased muscle or joint pain, decreased swelling in your hands and feet, fewer headaches, improved gastrointestinal symptoms (diarrhea, gas, nausea, stomach pain), improved sleep, less anxiety, stress and/or brain fog, less bloating, lower blood sugar, more energy, fewer cravings, and weight loss. Then start to reintroduce those foods back into your diet one at a time, waiting three to seven days between each food initiation. You can then evaluate whether you have a reaction to bringing them back into your diet. As you reintroduce foods, watch for changes in your digestion, energy, sleep, cravings, mood, behavior, skin, breathing, pain and inflammation, and medical conditions or symptoms.

START SOMEWHERE

My last thought on focusing on your fork is to simply start—somewhere. Making sweeping dietary changes all at once is overwhelming and usually ineffective. Instead, start by making some gradual changes. Although my intention for this book is not to focus on one's weight, it is common for my clients to seek out my advice when trying to achieve a more ideal body weight or to maintain their ideal weight. My recommendations are to:

- Remember moderation.
- Get your calories in check by tracking if you are eating and drinking in excess of your maintenance.
- Eat a low-glycemic breakfast, high in protein and low in starch, to stabilize your blood sugar for the rest of the day.
- SWAP high glycemic foods with low glycemic foods when possible.
- Consume 1–2 cups of veggies with meals.
- Aim to hit 20–30 grams of protein at meals and snacks.
- Focus on your fiber intake by getting a minimum of 25–38 grams per day (women to men respectively).
- Consume less than 2,400 mg of sodium and under 9.5 teaspoons of sugar daily.
- Track your steps and increase your daily steps if needed. Shoot for 8–10K steps per day on a weekly average, with 3–4 moderate to vigorous intensity workouts per week that consist of progressive strength training.

- Stay consistent even if you do not lose weight every week.
- Focus on ways to optimize your metabolism instead of eating significantly below your caloric needs.
- Add a multivitamin and multimineral that includes all the Bs, vitamin D3 + K2, omega-3 supplement, magnesium (magnesium glycinate if you are not constipated, magnesium citrate if you are), and probiotic with a prebiotic to your daily regimen.

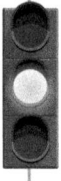

YELLOW LIGHT MOMENT

Turn to **Worksheet H**. It is time for your Yellow Light Moment. Ask yourself:

- How can I optimize my nutrition?
- What golden nuggets did I take away from this chapter?
- What can I start to implement immediately to improve the quality and value of my food?

Write 3 action steps and start to implement at least 1 of them this week.

CHAPTER 5

Self-Care Is A Necessity

I AM GIVING YOU PERMISSION right now to turn down the noise in your life. Soften the space between your eyebrows, let your shoulders drop and relax your back, unclench your jaw, drop your tongue from the roof of your mouth, take a deep breath in, exhale slowly, and simply surrender while you melt into this moment.

Your mental and emotional health is vital to your quality of life and day-to-day experience. When it comes to achieving long-term health and vitality, how we treat ourselves and manage all aspects of our stress is too often a neglected part of our lives. We live in a modern world where the pace, noise, expectations, information overload, and interruptions challenge us daily. We are overstressed, overstimulated, and overcommitted. Your fatigue is real. Your exhaustion is real. Feeling overwhelmed is real. Do not feel guilty about needing breaks in your daily life. When we are faced with acute stress, our bodies pump out adrenaline and cortisol necessary for a fight-or-flight response. Consider this... when stress occurs, even if you imagine it, your body reacts—it will either fight for your life or run for your life. Your blood thickens, your heart rate increases, your energy spikes with a flood of glucose into your bloodstream, and your mind sharpens. This is a great system if you are truly in a unique stressful, need-to-survive situation. But what about when this is caused by everyday stress? This type of chronic stress is wreaking havoc on our bodies as our stress hormone, cortisol, remains elevated in our system due to our diets, traumas, isolation, jobs, schedules, and stressors. Where is the pause? This is where taking a Yellow Light Moment in self-care becomes an essential player in maximizing your health and vitality.

Self-care means you are working to preserve and improve your own health, while also incorporating techniques and strategies to cope with and reduce stress, avoiding the continual elevation of cortisol in your system. This includes taking care of your emotional, spiritual, psychological, and social well-being. Chronic stress is linked to numerous deficits in your body. You experience mood swings, inability to concentrate, low energy levels, an increase in headaches, more breakouts, increased blood pressure, a decrease in the immune system, diarrhea, constipation, indigestion, stomach aches, loss of libido, changes in menstrual cycles, increased inflammation, and aches and pains in the joints and muscles. If you are in the habit of putting your self-care at the bottom of the priority list, I strongly encourage you to reassess that practice.

Sometimes you need to take a step back and learn how to say "no." You need to ask for help. You need to spend time alone or you need to surround yourself with a support system. You need to put yourself first. You need to set boundaries. You need to know what reenergizes you. Self-care is not selfish; your mental health is a priority because if you do not take care of yourself, it will spill over into every aspect of your life—from personal relationships to professional efficiency.

Get in the habit of asking yourself the following questions:

- Am I feeling off?
- When was the last time I drank water?
- When was the last time I ate something nourishing?
- When was the last time I got up and walked around?
- When was the last time I went outside to get fresh air?
- When was the last time I took time for myself to disconnect?
- When was the last time I connected with others?

- When was the last time I stopped to get clarity and ask if I felt that I was in alignment?
- When was the last time I felt centered and at peace?

MINDFULNESS

Self-care involves taking deliberate actions to protect, prioritize, and enhance your physical, mental, spiritual, and emotional well-being. One of the ways to accomplish this is to practice mindfulness. Mindfulness helps manage stress by keeping you present in the moment. Chances are you have heard about mindfulness, even if you did not truly know how to explain it. This ancient practice is beneficial to nearly every part of your life. It is a mental state characterized by being fully present and engaged in the current moment—without judgment or distraction. It involves paying attention to your thoughts and feelings—without being overwhelmed by them or reacting to them impulsively. Imagine focusing on the present moment and being fully engaged in your current experience. Imagine being conscious of your thoughts and feelings—without being consumed by them. Imagine accepting thoughts and feelings—without labeling them as good or bad. Imagine acknowledging things as they are—without the need to change them, but rather accepting the reality of the present moment.

How mindful are you? Ask yourself:

- Do I experience emotions without realizing them until later?
- Do I frequently miss details of my day because I am thinking about something else?
- Do I walk and drive so fast that I fail to experience and appreciate what I am passing?
- Do I forget people's names as soon as I meet them?
- Do I feel I am running on autopilot all the time?
- Do I find myself listening to someone while thinking of something else?
- Do I think of the future without being present in the moment?
- Do I eat without being hungry or tasting my food?

You can practice mindfulness by incorporating yoga, meditating, praying, or reframing a negative thought with a positive one. Find something you appreciate most in your life—playing music, going outside for a walk, completing guided imagery, repeating a mantra, journaling, and even coloring. This gives you time to step back from your emotions, stay present, in the moment, break the cycle of worry and stress, and decide what is important to you instead of simply reacting to situations.

Research shows that practicing mindfulness can have numerous positive effects on your health. It lowers stress hormone levels by training your body and brain not to enter fight-or-flight mode. Instead, now you remain calmer under pressure and do not overreact as quickly. It focuses your attention, decreases depression, reduces inflammation, and boosts your immune system. Each time you practice mindfulness, you practice not reacting, instead inserting a pause into a behavioral cascade, helping to override emotional impulses.

Try it right now. After you read the rest of this paragraph set your alarm for 3–5 minutes. Turn off your devices or silence them. Close your eyes. Listen to your breath. Observe, without judgment, any thoughts that come and go from your mind. I bet you will feel better the moment you open your eyes again.

MINDFUL MOVES

Moving on autopilot is not the ideal way to move through life. Here are a few more techniques to build mindfulness and practice self-care. You can better manage your stress throughout the day as you work to recharge your mind, body, and soul.

Take a Digital Detox

Remember how I said in Chapter 3 we seem to unplug by plugging in? How many of us grab our phones first thing in the morning, check it while having a meal or a snack, feel like we have lost a limb if we leave it at home while we run errands, sit on the couch while browsing the latest social feed instead of engaging in conversation with those around us, and lay in bed at night with the lights gleaming into our eyes? We have not learned to regulate our relationships with these devices. Although they are extremely helpful tools in our lives, they can also cause a stress-filled digital overload. When needing to disconnect from phones, computers, tablets, or anything adding a digital feed, consider the following strategies:

- When you wake up in the morning resist the urge to roll over and grab your phone or digital device. After your alarm goes off take 3–5 deep breaths and stretch out while you are still lying flat in bed. Now let your day begin. You can take this a step further and make your bedroom a device-free zone. This ensures you will not be grabbing it first thing in the morning. A regular alarm clock will do the trick waking you.
- Turn off notifications during the day on your phone and your smartwatch for anyone or anything nonessential. This nonstop pinging disrupts your focus.
- Designate some digital-free time. This is a perfect way to disconnect from the devices, and to be more present at work, and for the people and experiences around you.
- Put away your phone, tablets, and computers while you are on vacation. Set up an automated response to emails and phone messages letting people know you "will return their message as soon as you can, in the order it was received because they are important to you." This will let others know you have heard them, but have set boundaries, and are unavailable enjoying your experience away from the digital world.
- Unsubscribe from all unnecessary email lists.

Challenge: Do you know you can set your phone up to notify you any time you have more than a particular number of pickups or a certain accumulation of screen time in a day? I am not denying how amazing these little electronic devices are, but I do believe we need to understand the magnitude of using them and be more mindful regarding the amount of time spent on them. This week, challenge yourself to check your pickups and screen times and assess if you need to evaluate the amount of time connected to your devices.

Meditation

Meditation is a practice that involves training the mind to achieve a state of mental clarity, relaxation, and heightened awareness. It has been practiced for thousands of years in various cultures and religions around the world. It helps to reduce stress, improve focus, and heighten your emotional well-being, mind-body connection, and spiritual growth. While there are numerous meditation techniques, most share some common elements, such as focused attention, controlled breathing, and a quiet environment. A few of the most common meditation techniques include mindfulness, transcendental, loving-kindness, and guided. *Mindfulness meditation* involves paying attention to the present moment without judgement. This often involves focusing on the breath or observing sensations in the body. *Transcendental meditation* is a form of silent meditation that involves repeating a mantra to achieve a state of relaxed awareness and stress relief. *Loving-kindness meditation* focuses on developing feelings of compassion and love toward oneself and others. *Guided meditation* involves following the guidance of a teacher or recorded audio to lead you through a specific meditation.

How to start your meditation:

1. Find a quiet and comfortable place where you will not be disturbed.
2. Sit or lie down in a comfortable position. There is no one-size-fits-all posture, the key is to be relaxed and alert.
3. Choose a point of focus, such as your breath, a mantra, or a visual object.
4. Start with a few minutes and gradually increase as you become more comfortable with the practice.

Like any skill, meditation improves with regular practice. Consistency is more important than duration. It is also a personal practice, and there is no right or wrong way to do it. It is about finding what works best for you. If you are new to meditation, you may find it helpful to explore different techniques and resources to discover what resonates best with you.

Try my favorite shower meditation: in the shower focus on the sensation of the warm water flowing over your body. Close your eyes and listen to the sound of the water hitting the shower floor, visualize the water washing away your negative thoughts, stress, and anxiety. Let your thoughts, beliefs, and feelings that no longer serve you, wash down the drain. Take a deep breath and enjoy the aroma of the soap. Start to feel lighter and much clearer.

Morning Vitality 5-Minute Mindset

Take five minutes to set yourself up for success today by prioritizing what is most important. When there is an abundance of tasks on your To-Do List, somehow, the most important things that need your attention and have the biggest return on investment physically, emotionally, and mentally can fall to the bottom of that list, while everything else rises to the top. Right now, I want you to focus on the three most essential tasks for your health and wellness and then let the rest go. These are the three biggest items—if you were to accomplish them today, they would make the greatest impact on your life. Now that you have these three things in your mind, I want you to imagine going through your day with them as the priority. Imagine yourself refocusing, saying no to all those other things that come along, and instead saying yes to your top three priorities. Picture what today will look like and how it will feel to put up some boundaries around everything else that is not serving your health and wellness goals. Now to make sure that you are going to start off on the right foot, I want you to imagine what the next hour of your life will look like. What are the immediate next steps you are going to take to make today your best day? Make it a **great** day!

Prayer

Prayer is a practice that involves a conversation with a divine being or higher power. It is a way to express your thoughts, feelings, gratitude, requests, or simply foster a sense of connection. A very personal act, prayer can take several forms—the spoken word, silent thoughts, meditation, rituals, or traditions. There are many benefits of praying. Engaging in prayer can have a calming effect on the mind and body, helping to reduce stress, anxiety, and promoting a sense of inner peace, hope, and optimism.

Prayer also involves reflection on your thoughts, actions, and beliefs. This reflective process can lead to increased self-awareness and personal growth. Participating in communal prayer can also foster a sense of belonging and community.

Incorporating prayer into your daily routine can be achieved by following these steps:

- **Set a Time:** Choose a consistent time each day to devote to prayer, whether it's in the morning, before bed, or during a break in your day.
- **Create a Sacred Space:** Designate a quiet and peaceful area where you can pray without distractions. This could be a corner of your room, a garden, or a cozy spot by a window.
- **Choose Prayer Format:** Decide on the type of prayer you want to engage in, whether it's traditional prayers, spontaneous prayers, meditation, or journaling.
- **Start Small:** Begin with a manageable duration for your prayer practice, gradually increasing it as it becomes a habit.
- **Use Reminders:** Set alarms or reminders on your phone or place visual cues in your environment to prompt you to pray at your chosen time.
- **Select Prayer Resources:** Gather prayer books, scripture passages, or devotional materials that resonate with you and incorporate them into your practice.
- **Practice Gratitude:** Begin or end your prayer with expressions of gratitude, acknowledging blessings and moments of grace in your life.
- **Stay Flexible:** Be open to adjusting your prayer routine to fit your evolving needs and circumstances, allowing for spontaneity and creativity in your practice. Prayer can happen anywhere at any time!
- **Stay Consistent:** Commit to your daily prayer ritual, even on days when you don't feel like it. Consistency is key to establishing prayer as an integral part of your daily life.
- **Reflect and Adapt:** Take time to reflect on the impact of prayer on your life and adjust your practice as needed to deepen your connection with the divine and nurture your spiritual growth.

Take a "Coffee Break"
As you are preparing your coffee in the morning (or tea, lemon water, bone broth... insert your drink of choice) take a minute to think about your intention for the day and visualize what a successful day will look like. Have gratitude for the day ahead of you and start your day with a positive mindset. Say a few positive affirmations and direct the narrative for your day—this can replace negative thought patterns and boost your self-confidence.

Catch Some Rays
Enjoy the sunshine and strive to get at least fifteen minutes of sunlight every morning, ideally within thirty minutes of waking up. It is a great time to connect with the sun, the fresh air, and the outdoors. Close your eyes and focus on the light trying to come into your eyes, feel the air temperature on your face, and smell the nature around you.

Enjoy the Scenery
On your commute (if you have one), whether it is driving, bicycling, walking, or taking public transportation, try to be present and not act out of habit. Many times, we arrive at our destination without remembering how we got there. Learn to take in the sights and appreciate the scenery around you. Use your commute as a time for meditation or mindfulness exercises while you focus on your breath and try to clear your mind.

Stop Multitasking
While at work focus on not multitasking. Time chunk (definition below!) your day in order to work on one task at a time. Keep one browser open at a time. Eat your meals away from your desk. Check your emotions occasionally at work. It is good to know if you need to take a break from what you are doing or a few deep breaths to reset yourself.

Time chunking, also known as time blocking or block scheduling, is a time-management technique that involves breaking your day into chunks, or blocks of time, and dedicating them to specific tasks or activities. The idea is to focus on one type of activity during each designated time block, rather than constantly switching between different tasks. This approach can help improve productivity, concentration, and overall time-management skills. By dedicating a specific block of time to a particular task or type of work, you can immerse yourself solely in that activity without the distraction of other tasks. Knowing that you have a set time to work on a specific task can also reduce procrastination. It encourages you to start and complete tasks within the allocated time limits. Time chunking requires planning and prioritization and increases awareness to identify situations where you may be wasting time, or situations where you could be more efficient. Use **Worksheet I: Time Chunking Your Day** and see how this time-management technique can work for you.

Feel Your Fingerprints

Have you ever taken the time to slow down and feel your fingerprints? Take a second right now to close your eyes and lightly rub your thumb and index finger together to feel the ridges in your fingerprints. Then switch to your thumb and middle finger, thumb and ring finger, and finally thumb and pinky. Slow your breathing and focus on the sensation. Now take this moment to a broader scale and complete a body scan starting at the top of your head, down your neck and shoulders, your chest, arms, hands, fingers, stomach, hips, thighs, knees, calves, and feet.

Move Your Body

During your workout, staying centered could lead to better results and more appreciation for moving your body. Do not rush through your workout just to get it done but enjoy the sense of satisfaction for a job well done. Yes, sometimes we want to zone out during a workout and that can be meditative, but if you are too distracted you could lose connection to what you are doing. Start by having a purpose for each workout. Are you there to complete your planned workout, strengthen specific muscles, challenge yourself during an interval, or dedicate the time to a positive mindset? Focus on the beat of your music, the words of your podcast, the sound of the machines, or the movement and feeling of your muscles. Be aware of your surroundings and focus on the magnificent work you are doing for your body, mind, and soul. You do not have to focus your entire workout on a state of awareness but try to focus on building awareness for 3–5 minutes and then decide if you want to increase the time from there.

Appreciate Your Food
While you are preparing dinner, take time to touch, smell, and look at all the ingredients of your meal. Mindfully put together a well-balanced plate and find gratitude in how it will nourish your body. Take time to eat your meal slowly, without distractions. Turn off the TV. Place your phone in another room. Take smaller bites and chew your food slowly. Place your fork down between bites. Savor each bite as you smell it and truly taste the flavors and textures. Drink water during your meal. Tune into your body and ask yourself halfway through your meal if you are still hungry or if you are at a point where you could stop eating. Also, acknowledge your feelings about, or responses to, various foods without judgment. Ask yourself if you are continuing to eat because of stress or emotion of the day.

Journaling
Journaling is a personal and reflective practice of regularly expressing your thoughts and feelings—often in a diary, notebook, or journal. Journaling exists in various forms, including—free writing, following structured prompts, listing bullet points, or even through artistic expressions such as drawings, scribbles, or collages. By putting thoughts on paper and dedicating a space for self-reflection, you can gain insights into your emotions, behaviors, and patterns of thinking. This can lead to personal growth and better understanding of yourself. Journaling may also serve as a healthy outlet for feelings of joy, anger, sadness, frustration, pride, peace, or confusion. This emotional release can contribute to improved mental and emotional well-being as you process your feelings and emotions. The process can also be a therapeutic tool for managing stress. By writing about stressful events or challenging situations, you may find a sense of relief and gain a clearer perspective of a situation. It can also help organize your thoughts and identify practical solutions to problems. Journaling can be a powerful tool for acknowledging setbacks and tracking personal goals. By documenting aspirations, progress, obstacles, and failures, you can stay focused, motivated, and accountable. It's a great habit that can enhance your goal achievement and personal development. Some people also use journaling to foster creativity. Whether through writing, drawing, or brainstorming, the act of transferring ideas to paper can stimulate your

imagination and help you explore new perspectives. Journals are also used to cultivate a sense of gratitude by regularly noting things for which you are thankful. This practice can contribute to a positive mindset and overall contentment in your life.

Here are a few journaling prompts to get you started:

- List three things you are grateful for today.
- Describe what you will let go of today.
- Reflect on a person who recently left a positive mark on your life.
- What are your current thoughts and feelings?
- Describe a challenging situation you recently faced and how you handled it.
- Describe a moment when you felt completely present and engaged.
- Reflect on a recent accomplishment and acknowledge your efforts.
- Recount a cherished childhood memory.
- Describe a recent experience that brought you joy.
- Describe how you have practiced self-care today.
- Reflect on a mistake you made, and the lessons you learned.
- Draw or doodle in your journal to visually express yourself.
- Describe a place you dream of visiting and why it appeals to you.
- Write a letter to your future self, outlining your aspirations and dreams.
- Write a letter to your younger self, offering advice and encouragement.

Use **Worksheet J: Yellow Light Moment Journal Page** or **Worksheet K: Blank Journal Page** to take a Yellow Light Moment and share your reflections and observations.

Mantra

Repeating a mantra can help you find your place of calm and clarity. A mantra can be a word, a sound, or a phrase that you repeat several times to feel connected, manage stress, cultivate a positive mindset, and invite stillness. The power is in finding one that speaks to you. It might take some experimentation as you try it out. Here are a few examples if you need help getting started:

- I am blessed.
- I love being me.
- Let it be.
- Be here, right now.
- I am at peace.
- Breathe in, breathe out.
- I can do this.
- I am limitless.
- It's going to be ok.

Do you have a mantra that speaks to you? Write it here in the blank space of this page or jot a few of them down on **Worksheet L: Writing Your Mantra** in the back of this book.

Deep Breathing

We spend our entire lives breathing so why do we find it hard to get a good breath some days? Deep breathing activates the body's relaxation response, aiding in stress reduction and anxiety management. Deep breathing exercises often involve mindfulness and conscious awareness of your breath. This can help clear your mind, regulate emotions, and improve your concentration. Incorporating deep breathing into your daily routine, especially during stressful or challenging moments, can contribute to your overall sense of well-being and improve both physical and mental health. It is a simple, yet powerful practice that can be done almost anywhere, making it accessible for individuals of all ages and fitness levels.

There are four types of breathing:

- **Eupnea breathing** occurs when you are not thinking about it, it is also referred to as quiet or unlabored breathing, so as you are reading this right now, I would assume you are probably using this type.

- **Diaphragmatic breathing**, known as deep breathing or belly breathing, occurs when you consciously use your diaphragm to take deep breaths.
- **Costal breathing** is shallow breathing, also known as chest breathing and is usually associated with stress.
- **Hyperpnea** is known as forced breathing, in which inhalation and exhalation are both forced. It usually happens when you exercise or when you are doing something strenuous.

Let's focus further on diaphragmatic (deep) breathing. It is important because it:

- helps you relax as it activates the parasympathetic nervous system (PNS) which is our rest and digest system, as opposed to our sympathetic nervous system (SNS) which is tied to fight or flight;
- activates the vagus nerve, which is the heavy hitter of the PNS, controlling things like our mood, digestion, and heart rate;
- can help with anxiety, depression, managing stress, improving focus, better sleep, and recovery from exercise or exertion;
- increases how much oxygen is in your blood.

Diaphragmatic breathing utilizes the diaphragm, which is a dome shaped muscle located at the base of your lungs. If you are breathing correctly, it will contract and move downward so your lungs can expand to take in fresh air. When you exhale, the diaphragm relaxes and slides further up into your chest cavity. Try practicing diaphragmatic breathing like this:

- Lie on your back on a flat surface with your knees bent and your head supported. You can use a pillow under your knees to support your legs.
- Place one hand on your upper chest and the other just below your rib cage.
- Breathe in slowly through your nose, so that your stomach moves out, causing your hand to rise. The hand on your chest should remain as still as possible.

- Tighten your stomach muscles, so that your stomach moves in, causing your hand to lower as you exhale, similar to blowing up a balloon.
- Repeat this 3–5 times.
- Practice this diaphragmatic breathing for 5–10 minutes about 3–4 times per day.

There are many different breathing exercises you can incorporate into your daily routine. One recommended breathing technique is **Alternate Nostril Breathing.** In this technique, you will take turns inhaling through one nostril and exhaling through the other. Here's how:

- Start by sitting up straight.
- Close your right nostril with your right thumb while inhaling through your left nostril.
- Now close your left nostril with your ring finger so both nostrils are held closed for a moment, then open your right nostril and exhale slowly through it.
- Next inhale through your right nostril, then hold both nostrils closed with your ring finger and thumb.
- Open your left nostril and exhale slowly through your left side.
- Repeat 5–10 times.

Box Breathing is also known as square breathing. It is a simple and effective relaxation technique that gets its name from the idea of visualizing a box or square as a pattern. Try this:

- Find a comfortable position and relax your shoulders.
- Close your eyes to help you focus and eliminate external distractions.
- Inhale slowly and deeply through your nose counting to four.
- After inhaling, hold your breath for a count of four. Keep the air in your lungs without straining.
- Exhale slowly and completely through your mouth, counting to four.
- Pause and hold your breath for another count of four.
- Repeat this cycle for 2–3 minutes, allowing tension to release with each cycle.

Relaxation Techniques

Progressive Muscle Relaxation (PMR) is a relaxation technique that was developed by Edmund Jacobson in the 1920s. This technique involves tensing and then gradually releasing different muscle groups in the body. It's a method commonly used to reduce stress and anxiety, promote relaxation, and improve sleep. To practice progressive muscle relaxation, first find a quiet and restful environment where you will not be disturbed. Next, get comfortable by sitting or lying down. Focus on breathing by taking a few deep breaths to relax your body and clear your mind. Start with a specific muscle group. Tense the muscle in that group for five to ten seconds, then release the tension suddenly. Pay attention to the sensations of tension and relaxation. Progress through different muscle groups in a systematic manner: hands and forearms, biceps and upper arms, face, neck and shoulders, chest and upper back, abdomen, glutes, thighs, calves, and feet. As you tense and release each muscle group, focus on the sensations of tension leaving your body, resulting in the feeling of relaxation that quickly takes over. Keep the rest of your body as relaxed as possible while you work on each muscle group. You can repeat the process if needed or spend more time on specific areas that feel particularly tense. Practice mindfulness by staying present and focused on the sensations in each muscle group. For the best results, make PMR a regular routine. Daily practice can help train your body to relax more easily.

Learn to Say "No"

Feeling the need to take a Yellow Light Moment is one few of us are immune to. We are bombarded with increasing options, opportunities, and obligations of a "just one more" society. One more... activity, committee, engagement, social hour, decision, expectation, meeting, carpool, practice, purchase, errand, question, email, text, etc. We all have a point where our "just one more" exceeds our physical, emotional, and mental ability—leading to overloading our system and ending with a breakdown of pure exhaustion. We need to understand that everyone has a different breaking point. We all must draw the line and set limits by taking the effort and the ability to say "no." It is not rude, insensitive, or selfish, it is a necessity. I do not say "no" because I am so busy, I say "no" because I do not want to be so busy. Remember to reflect on your values and priorities at times like these. Knowing what is truly important to you can make it easier to decline requests that do not align with your goals. Practice being assertive and clearly expressing your thoughts and feelings. Learn to pause before responding, to protect your time and your energy, and know it is okay to say no without giving a reason. "No" is a complete sentence.

When learning to say no or deciding what you are willing to let go of, consider the following prompts:

- Does this align with my values and long-term goals?
- Will saying yes add unnecessary stress or overwhelm to my schedule?
- Is this request more important than my current commitments?
- Am I agreeing out of guilt or obligation rather than genuine desire?
- How will this impact my well-being and mental health?
- Is there someone else who can handle this better or more efficiently?
- What are the potential consequences of saying no versus saying yes?
- Do I have the time and energy to give this my best effort?
- Will this opportunity or commitment help me grow or add value to my life?
- How often have I said yes recently, and do I need to rebalance my priorities?

Here's a guide to help you identify and articulate these changes in the areas of sleep, nutrition, self-care, and movement **Worksheet M: Saying "No."**

Create White Space

Avoid overloading your schedule with too many tasks. Work on setting realistic and achievable goals to prevent overwhelming chaos, but also remember no matter how well you plan, life happens. Make room for it by leaving space in your schedule for the unexpected. This helps you from overextending your energy when those obstacles do arise. Leave gaps for spontaneity, time to process before the next appointment, or just quiet brain time to recharge. Regularly assess your schedule and adjust it as needed. If you find yourself consistently overwhelmed, consider reevaluating your priorities and making the necessary changes.

Express Yourself

Express yourself through art, music, dance, or any creative outlet. Engage in activities that you enjoy. This will provide a joyous mental break from stressors; one you will look forward to doing. Pursue hobbies that bring you a sense of accomplishment and relaxation. Take a class you have been wanting to sign up for, contact a professional about taking lessons, or create a designated space in your home to support your activity.

Get a Massage

Getting a massage can offer a wide range of physical, mental, and emotional benefits. It can promote relaxation and reduce stress levels by triggering the release of endorphins. A massage can target specific muscles or muscle groups, to help alleviate tension and reduce pain. It can enhance blood flow by improving the delivery of oxygen and nutrients to the muscles and other tissues. It can help increase flexibility and improve range of motion. A massage is valuable for individuals involved in physical activities or those recovering from injuries. It can promote better sleep. A massage can stimulate the lymphatic system, aiding in the removal of waste products and toxins from the body, among other potential benefits.

Declutter Your Spaces

Decluttering is not just about creating a visually appealing space; it is about promoting a healthier and more balanced lifestyle. Clutter can be overwhelming and contribute to and increase your stress and anxiety levels. A tidy and organized space promotes a sense of serenity and order. It also allows you to concentrate on tasks more effectively because you will be less likely to be distracted by the visual noise of clutter. Set aside specific times for decluttering to avoid feeling overwhelmed. Whether it's 15 minutes a day or an hour each weekend, having a schedule helps you stay consistent and make steady progress. Go through your space, room by room, and donate or trash anything that is not a favorite or necessary item. See **Worksheet N: 28 Days To Declutter Your Home Checklist.**

Pay Attention to Your Joy

Your true joy is the direct opposite of triggers that increase your stress. There are moments, even when small, that true joy brings peace, connection, and calmness to your life. These things make you feel rejuvenated, energized, uplifted, and happy. Once you start looking for them you will see them more frequently. Find moments that bring ease, bonds that feel safe, people who bring togetherness, situations that bring warmth, relationships that feel like a hug, individuals who bring understanding, and feelings that show love. Then work to increase those things and moments in your life.

Build Social Connections

When you feel like you belong and you have the support, attention, and care you need in the quality of relationships you want, you have found your community. This group, who are "your people," offer emotional support, practical help, and advice resulting in decreased feelings of stress and isolation. This connectedness is important for our psychological well-being to belong to something larger than ourselves. You can foster positive relationships and expand your social connections by—joining a group or club, volunteering your time, reconnecting with a classmate, sending a brief text to your bestie, signing up to take a new class, hosting a dinner party, inviting a friend to grab a cup of coffee, asking a neighbor to go for a walk, and sharing lunch with a co-worker.

Protect Your Energy

Your energy is guided by the people you surround yourself with, the way you spend your time, the books you read, the content you consume, the food you eat, the words you speak to yourself, the movement you take, the relaxation you prioritize, the work you do on yourself, the kindness you show yourself, the self-forgiveness you encourage, the boundaries you set, and the way you show up for yourself. Learn to protect your energy.

Laugh

Find humor in everyday life. Laughter is a natural stress reliever. When you laugh, your body releases endorphins—neurotransmitters that promote an overall sense of well-being that can temporarily relieve pain. The act of laughing also reduces the levels of stress hormones like cortisol, leading to a more relaxed state. Shared laughter helps strengthen social bonds and builds a sense of community and connection among people. It enhances relationships, whether among friends, family, or colleagues. Laughter has positive effects on the cardiovascular system by improving blood flow and promoting a healthy heart, boosting the immune system by increasing the production of immune cells and antibodies. It has also been associated with improving respiratory function and increasing lung capacity. Laughter triggers the release of neurotransmitters like dopamine and serotonin, our happy hormones, associated with—pleasure, calmness, and mood elevation—providing a healthy perspective on life. Seek out funny movies and shows, listen to humorous podcasts, go to a comedy club, and spend time with people who genuinely make you laugh.

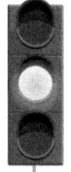

YELLOW LIGHT MOMENT

Turn to **Worksheet O**. It is time for your Yellow Light Moment. Ask yourself:

- How can I optimize my self-care?
- What golden nuggets did I take away from this chapter?
- What can I start to implement immediately to improve the quality and quantity of my self-care?

Write 3 action steps and start to implement at least 1 of them this week.

CHAPTER 6

Movement Is Key

DO YOU WANT to know what I personally and professionally believe to be the absolute best workout program for you? Whatever you will do consistently, day in and day out, without fail, for the rest of your life! Stop starting over. Find what works for *you* and do it. Set a movement goal every day! Not everyone gets the same adrenaline rush and high endorphin release from a good sweat session at the gym, so I want to encourage you to find something you enjoy that helps you feel energized and refreshed. Choose something that increases your movement, muscle, and mobility. Stop making excuses for why you are not working out and start realizing that negotiating your way out of your next workout is a choice. Remember inaction is still an action. You must become your own disciplinarian and commit to your success.

I know you probably thought I was going to lead this book with exercise because I am a gym owner and personal trainer. And yes—I absolutely do believe that exercise is the most underutilized anti-depressant, and that movement must be a daily event in your life. But when you are exhausted, malnourished, and over-stressed your workouts will not be your best. Most likely you will skip them altogether because of those very things. This is why you need to balance the equation of sleep, nutrition, and self-care along with movement. When finding how to increase your movement pause and ask yourself:

- What challenges me?
- What makes me feel confident and strong?
- What type of exercise am I most consistent with?
- What do I enjoy doing?

Use **Worksheet P: Movement Questionnaire** to write down your answers.

Is your ideal movement scenario having a personal trainer who is going to write your routines and help you with form and follow through? Maybe it's attending a group fitness class with your neighbor or friend so you have someone to call you out when you do not show up (yes, your trainer will do that too). Perhaps you feel more comfortable with a quiet yoga session, a virtual class at your convenience, training with a specific goal set for an upcoming event, or a mix of all the above? You do you! At the end of the day, it is exactly that—*you* against *you*. You are becoming a better version of yourself for you. If you cannot seem to find your groove or feel you are in a rut, then be creative and try lots of different things. Get on a bike, go for a swim, hike in nature, start a walk-to-run program, buy a kayak, learn to row, try hot yoga, get on a ski machine, or pick up some free weights. Every bit of movement helps. For example, a single session of moderate-to-vigorous physical activity can reduce blood pressure, improve insulin sensitivity, improve sleep, reduce anxiety symptoms, and improve some aspects of cognition on the day that it is performed.[14] The end goal is to address all five elements of fitness: cardiorespiratory endurance, muscle strength, muscle endurance, flexibility, and body composition by creating a fitness plan that incorporates these elements, ensuring you get the most health benefits from your routine.

---

[14] Physical Activity Guidelines for Americans, 2nd Ed. 2018. U.S. Department of Health and Human Services.

FIVE ELEMENTS OF FITNESS

Before we dive into the five elements of fitness, it is important to talk about safety when starting a physical activity. Begin by consulting your healthcare professional about the types and amounts of activity that are appropriate for you. This is especially true if you suffer from a chronic condition or experience symptoms related to one. Next, choose an activity that is appropriate for your current level of fitness and your health goals. If you are a beginner, start with a lower intensity activity and gradually increase how often and how long each activity should be done. Understand that with all activities there are risks involved, so protect yourself with the appropriate gear and choose safe environments in regard to where and when you should be active. Special recommendations are often offered for children, older adults, women who are pregnant or postpartum, or adults with chronic diseases or with disabilities.

Now let us explore the five elements to include when building a workout program.

Cardiorespiratory Endurance

Cardiorespiratory endurance, also known as aerobic fitness or cardiovascular fitness, is the efficiency of the cardiovascular and respiratory systems. This aerobic conditioning focuses on the ability of the circulatory and respiratory systems to deliver and use oxygen. Aerobic exercise uses oxygen to fuel physical activity over a prolonged period of time. Your body needs to take oxygen and efficiently and effectively deliver it to your body's tissues through the heart, lungs, arteries, vessels, and veins. You must understand that no two individuals will ever respond and adapt to cardiorespiratory exercise in the same way. Therefore, when determining what program is right for you, take into consideration the frequency, intensity, time, type, and enjoyment of your program.

Frequency is the number of training sessions you are completing, usually expressed per week. For general health requirements the recommended frequency of activity is every day of the week, for small quantities of time. For improved fitness levels, the frequency is three to five days per week at higher intensities.

Intensity refers to the level of demand that a given activity places on your body. This can be evaluated in several ways—such as calculating heart rate, VO_2max which is the maximal oxygen consumption, or VO_2R which is the oxygen uptake reserve. The rating of perceived exertion, also known as the Borg Scale, is a subjective measurement to express your intensity of an exercise. Perceived exertion is based on the type of activity you are doing, how much your heart rate has increased, how much you are sweating, and how much muscle fatigue you are feeling. For general health requirements, moderate intensity is preferred. Higher intensities are generally required for improvements in overall fitness and conditioning.

FIGURE 6-1: Rating of Perceived Exertion (Borg Scale)

6	No exertion at all
7	Extremely light
8	
9	Very light
10	
11	Light
12	
13	Somewhat hard
14	
15	Hard (heavy)
16	
17	Very hard
18	
19	Extremely hard
20	Maximal exertion

Time is the length of period you are performing the activity. Adults should accumulate 150 minutes of moderate intensity aerobic activity such as brisk walking every week or 75 minutes of vigorous intensity aerobic activity, like jogging or running every week, or an equivalent mix of moderate and vigorous intensity aerobic activity.

Type is the kind of physical activity you are performing. For an exercise to be considered aerobic, it should a) be rhythmic in nature, b) use large muscle groups, and c) be continuous in nature.[15] Examples include running or jogging, brisk walking, exercising on cardio equipment, swimming, and cycling.

Enjoyment is exactly what it sounds like. How much joy are you getting from engaging in the exercise or activity you are completing? This last variable is important when trying to adhere to a program. It is important to note that a busy or active lifestyle or recreational activity is not always a substitute for cardiovascular exercise. You might feel you are on your feet all day long, walking here and there, and constantly on the go, but that movement does not always equate to exercise activity. Make sure your exercise is *intentional*. Running, brisk walking, cycling, swimming, dancing, rowing, boxing, and circuit training are a few intentional workouts.

WHY GO CARDIO?

There are numerous reasons to incorporate cardiorespiratory endurance into your routine. Let's begin with the most apparent one: your heart health. Regular cardiovascular exercise offers a multitude of benefits. To start, it strengthens the heart muscle, improves blood circulation, and helps reduce the risk of heart disease. This enhances the efficiency of the heart in pumping blood, which can result in lower blood pressure. Additionally, cardiorespiratory endurance boosts the efficiency of the respiratory system. This means the lungs can take in more oxygen and expel more carbon dioxide, improving overall respiratory function and capacity. Engaging in cardiovascular exercise aids in a reduction of calories, especially when combined with proper nutrition, promoting weight loss, and helping to prevent obesity-related conditions. Improved cardiorespiratory endurance also increases the body's ability to perform sustained, moderate-to-high-intensity activities without experiencing fatigue. This enhanced endurance and stamina are particularly beneficial for athletes and individuals involved in activities and occupations requiring prolonged exertion. Furthermore,

---

[15] Clark, Micheal A., Lucett, Scott C., and Sutton, Brian G., (2012) NASM Essentials of Personal Fitness Training. 4th Ed.

enhanced cardiorespiratory endurance aids quicker recovery by facilitating efficient oxygen delivery to muscles, and reducing the buildup of metabolic byproducts. Regular aerobic exercise has also been shown to boost energy levels and reduce feelings of fatigue. Additionally, it has been linked to the release of endorphins, which are the chemicals in the brain that act as natural mood lifters. Consistent activity can help alleviate symptoms of stress, anxiety, and depression while enhancing sleep quality and contributing to better immune function. There is evidence to suggest that individuals with higher levels of cardiorespiratory endurance tend to live longer and enjoy a higher quality of life in their later years.

Muscle Endurance and Muscle Strength

Muscle endurance and muscle strength are two factors that contribute to overall muscular health. For this reason, I am going to compare the two of them and then break them apart in this book. While muscular endurance measures the ability of a muscle or group of muscles to perform contractions over an extended period, muscular strength evaluates the maximum force a muscle or group of muscles can produce in one, all-out effort or your one-rep max.

Let's take a minute to just talk about muscle endurance. Muscle endurance is an essential component of overall fitness—it plays a key role in various aspects of daily life, sports performance, and overall health. It is vital for performing everyday tasks such as walking, climbing stairs, lifting groceries, and carrying out household chores. These are functional daily activities where having improved muscle endurance allows you to sustain these activities without fatigue. Outside of daily activities, many sports also require an elevated level of endurance. Activities like running, cycling, swimming, and team sports that involve repetitive moments over an extended period utilize muscle endurance. Your body is asked to perform the same movement again and again. This endurance also contributes to better joint stability and proper body mechanics, helping to prevent injuries by reducing the risk of muscle imbalances and fatigue. When you experience muscle imbalances and fatigue, your body may lose its proper form or start to compensate, which may result in injuries. Many activities that enhance muscle endurance can also provide cardiovascular benefits. They support overall metabolic health and help regulate blood sugar levels, improving insulin sensitivity. These activities help burn extra calories which is helpful in maintaining a healthy body weight or adding to a weight-management program.

Turn your attention now to muscle strength. You can imagine that muscular strength refers to the maximum amount of force a muscle or group of muscles can generate. There are many reasons this is important to your health and functionality. Muscle strength is essential for performing everyday activities such as lifting, carrying, pushing, and pulling. Having strong muscles improves your ability to complete these tasks with ease, while reducing the risk of injuries. You are able to perform your daily activities while also providing support to your joints, resulting in better joint stability. Muscular strength contributes to good posture by supporting the spine and aligning the body, properly maintaining a more upright and balanced position while preventing slouching. In sports and physical activities, muscular strength is often a key determinant of performance. Athletes who develop specific muscle groups related to their sport can improve their power, speed, and overall athletic abilities. Regular strength training has been associated with a reduced risk of chronic conditions such as heart disease, diabetes, and hypertension. It can positively impact various health markers—including blood pressure, cholesterol levels, and insulin sensitivity. Exercise, including strength training, has been linked to improved mood and reduced symptoms of anxiety and depression. Physical activity stimulates the release of endorphins—neurotransmitters that contribute to feeling of well-being. As you age, maintaining muscular strength is critical for keeping an independent lifestyle. Strong muscles support mobility, balance, and coordination, reducing the risk of falls—maintaining the ability to perform daily activities without assistance. Engaging in resistance training to build strong muscles also contributes to improved bone density. The stress placed on bones during strength training helps to maintain and enhance bone mass, reducing the risk of osteoporosis and fractures, especially as you increase in age. Muscles are metabolically active tissues, meaning they burn calories even at rest. Having more muscle mass can contribute to an increase in resting metabolic rate, aiding in weight management, and fat loss.

Resistance training, also referred to as strength training or weight training, is a form of exercise intended to increase both muscular strength and muscular endurance. This involves using various forms of resistance such as weights, bands, or your own body weight working against gravity. Notice I did not say you have to join a gym and learn Olympic lifting; you can get started with strength training using your own body weight to perform exercises like pushups, squats, and planks. You can also use common household items for your resistance. Grab weighted gallon jugs, water bottles filled with sand or rocks, or a backpack filled with books to use as your weights. By incorporating resistance, you can improve muscle strength and endurance, enhance speed and agility, boost metabolism, reduce body fat, increase bone density, improve balance and stability, and protect joints from injury. This training can lead to improved mental and emotional wellness helping alleviate depression symptoms and relieving general feelings of anxiety and worry, and increased self-esteem.

One of the most important things for you to remember during resistance training is how crucial it is that you use the proper form. This will ensure you are not only getting the most out of your workout, but that you are also decreasing your risk of injury. If you have been avoiding strength training because you are uncomfortable knowing where and how to start, this is a perfect time to contact a personal trainer who can design a program specifically for you and instruct you on proper form as you progress. The goal is to incorporate resistance training 2–3 days a week with various exercises that involve all the major muscle groups, as muscular endurance and muscular strength are body muscle group specific. This means it is possible for one area of your body to be stronger than another. For example, you could have strong biceps but weak hamstrings, or strong glutes and weak deltoids. Generally speaking, lifting heavier weights with fewer repetitions increases strength, taking your muscles to fatigue with each set; while lifting lighter weights with more repetitions increases endurance over time.

Flexibility

Flexibility is described as the ability to move a joint through its complete range of motion (ROM). This ROM is controlled by the normal extensibility, or ability to stretch, of all soft tissues surrounding the joint. Whether you are a weekend warrior, an elite athlete, or a 9–5 office employee, you need to add flexibility training to your program. Almost everyone can be affected by postural imbalances. Most of these imbalances are a result of too much sitting or too many repetitive movements. Your muscular and fascial systems are structured to function with a baseline of normal tension. However, it is common for normal tension to increase under conditions of mental and physical stress, sleep deficiency, dehydration, poor nutrition, physical deconditioning, decreased daily movement, and even just normal aging. Other factors that can influence your flexibility are your genetics, connective tissue elasticity, joint structure, body composition, sex, activity level, and any previous injuries. The good news is that adding flexibility training can improve muscle imbalances, increase joint ROM and muscle extensibility, relieve excessive tension of muscles and joint stress, and improve neuromuscular efficiency and function.

The best flexibility training programs incorporate multiple forms of stretching to be used before and after exercise or on recovery days. Here are a few I recommend:

SELF-MYOFASCIAL RELEASE
This technique involves applying gentle sustained pressure (such as with a foam roller) to areas that are tight or sore for a minimum of thirty seconds. This technique focuses on neuromuscular activation and can be used to warm up or cool down to reduce muscle tightness, soreness, and inflammation. It simultaneously helps improve your range of motion, increase blood flow, and aid in relaxation. Foam rollers are manufactured with different densities, surface textures (some are smooth while others have ridges or knobs), shapes, lengths, and diameters. I suggest starting with a low or medium density foam roller that is thirty-six inches long and six inches in diameter for versatile use.

One of my favorite areas to foam roll are my glutes. This helps relieve muscle tension, improve mobility, and enhance recovery. Here is a step-by-step guide to help you foam roll your glutes properly:

1. **Prepare Your Equipment**
   - Foam Roller: Choose a foam roller that suits your comfort level. Beginners may prefer a softer roller, while more experienced users might opt for a firmer one.
   - Space: Find an open, flat area with enough space to move around comfortably.
2. **Position Yourself on the Foam Roller**
   - Sit on the Roller: Start by sitting on the foam roller with your legs extended in front of you and your hands placed on the ground behind you for support.
   - Cross One Leg Over the Other: To target the right glute, cross your right ankle over your left knee. This will open up the glute muscle and allow for deeper rolling. Repeat the same for the left glute by crossing your left ankle over your right knee.
3. **Begin Rolling**
   - Lean Towards the Target Glute: Shift your body weight towards the glute you are rolling. For the right glute, lean slightly to the right, and for the left glute, lean to the left.
   - Roll Slowly: Begin to roll slowly from the top of your glute (near your lower back) to the bottom (near your hamstrings). Move in a controlled manner, rolling back and forth over the muscle.
4. **Identify Tight Spots**
   - Pause on Tender Areas: As you roll, you will likely encounter tender or tight spots. When you find these areas, pause, and hold for 30–60 seconds.
   - Breathe Deeply: Keep your breathing steady and deep while pausing on tight spots. This will help to relax the muscle and improve the effectiveness of the release.
5. **Adjust Your Position**
   - Change Angles: To fully work the glute muscles, adjust your body position slightly to roll at different angles. This ensures you cover the entire glute area, including the sides and upper portion near the hip.

- Switch Sides: After rolling one glute for about 1-2 minutes, switch to the other glute and repeat the process.
6. **Finish Up**
    - Stretch: After foam rolling, perform some gentle stretches to further relax and lengthen the glute muscles. A seated or lying glute stretch can be effective.
    - Hydrate: Drink water to help flush out any toxins released during the foam rolling process.
7. **Frequency and Duration**
    - Regular Routine: Incorporate foam rolling into your regular fitness routine. Aim to foam roll your glutes 3-4 times per week, or more often if you experience tightness or soreness.
    - Duration: Spend about 1-2 minutes per glute during each session, ensuring thorough coverage without overdoing it.
8. **Tips for Effective Foam Rolling**
    - Control Your Movement: Move slowly and deliberately to ensure you are effectively massaging the muscle.
    - Listen to Your Body: Foam rolling might be uncomfortable but should not be painful. If you experience sharp pain, stop immediately and consult a healthcare professional.
    - Use Your Core: Engage your core muscles to help control your movements and maintain stability.

STATIC STRETCHING

This technique involves taking a muscle to the point of tension without pain, and then passively holding that position for thirty seconds. This low force with longer duration stretch can be used before or after activity. Do not bounce into a stretch, but instead, hold it for a minimum of 30–60 seconds while performing static stretches. It is also important to keep a normal breath while holding a stretch. You should not hold your breath or feel pain, but you should feel tension in the stretch. Repeat the stretch 2-3 times during a stretch session. Aim to include static stretches in your routine several times a week.

Here are ten good static stretches that target different muscle groups throughout the body to enhance flexibility and reduce muscle tension:

1. **Hamstring Stretch**
   - Position: Sit on the floor with one leg extended straight and the other leg bent with the foot against the inner thigh of the extended leg.
   - Reach: Inhale and lengthen your spine, then exhale and slowly reach forward towards the toes of the extended leg. Keep your back straight.
   - Hold: Hold the stretch for 30–60 seconds, then switch legs.
2. **Quadriceps Stretch**
   - Position: Stand upright and balance on one leg. If needed, hold onto a wall or chair for support.
   - Pull: Bend your other knee and bring your heel towards your buttocks. Grab your ankle with your hand.
   - Hold: Keep your knees close together and hold the stretch for 30–60 seconds. Switch legs and repeat.
3. **Shoulder Stretch**
   - Position: Stand or sit up straight.
   - Cross: Bring one arm across your body at shoulder height.
   - Hold: Use your other hand to gently pull your arm closer to your chest. Hold the stretch for 30–60 seconds. Switch arms and repeat.
4. **Chest Stretch**
   - Position: Stand tall and clasp your hands behind your back.
   - Lift: Slowly lift your hands upwards, away from your back, while keeping your shoulders down and back.
   - Hold: Hold the stretch for 30–60 seconds. If needed, slightly bend forward at the hips to deepen the stretch.
5. **Calf Stretch**
   - Position: Stand facing a wall with your hands placed on the wall at shoulder height.
   - Step Back: Step one foot back, keeping the heel on the ground and the leg straight.
   - Bend Forward: Bend the front knee slightly and lean towards the wall until you feel a stretch in the calf of the back leg.
   - Hold: Hold the stretch for 30–60 seconds. Switch legs and repeat.

6. **Hip Flexor Stretch**
   - Position: Kneel on one knee with the other foot in front, creating a 90-degree angle at both knees.
   - Shift Forward: Gently shift your weight forward until you feel a stretch in the hip flexor of the back leg.
   - Hold: Hold the stretch for 30–60 seconds. Switch legs and repeat.
7. **Triceps Stretch**
   - Position: Stand or sit up straight.
   - Raise Arm: Raise one arm overhead, then bend the elbow to bring your hand behind your neck.
   - Pull: Use the opposite hand to gently push the elbow down and towards your head.
   - Hold: Hold the stretch for 30–60 seconds. Switch arms and repeat.
8. **Figure Four Glute Stretch**
   - Position: Lie on your back with your knees bent and feet flat on the floor.
   - Cross Ankle: Cross one ankle over the opposite knee, forming a figure four shape.
   - Pull: Gently pull the uncrossed leg towards your chest until you feel a stretch in the glutes.
   - Hold: Hold the stretch for 30–60 seconds. Switch legs and repeat.
9. **Child's Pose**
   - Position: Kneel on the floor, sit back on your heels, and extend your arms forward on the floor.
   - Reach Forward: Lower your torso between your knees, reaching your arms as far forward as comfortable.
   - Hold: Hold the stretch for 30–60 seconds, breathing deeply.
10. **Spinal Twist**
    - Position: Sit on the floor with your legs extended straight.
    - Bend Knee: Bend one knee and place the foot on the outside of the opposite thigh.
    - Twist: Twist your torso towards the bent knee, placing the opposite elbow on the outside of the bent knee for leverage.
    - Hold: Hold the stretch for 30–60 seconds, then switch sides.

DYNAMIC STRETCHING

This technique uses the force production of a muscle and the body's momentum to take a joint through a full range of motion. This active stretching can mimic the motion of sports specific repetitions you are about to start, thus, making it a good warmup before an athletic activity. Target different joints and muscles for 10–12 repetitions. For example, if you are a runner try leg pendulums (swinging each leg back and forth), walking lunges, and small hip circles.

Adequate flexibility when combined with exercise helps prevent injuries and contributes to good posture, allowing the body to maintain proper alignment as tight muscles can pull the body out of alignment, which over time can lead to musculoskeletal issues. This is also key for essential functional movements to perform daily activities with ease, such as reaching, bending, and turning. Your body is meant to move in a coordinated and efficient manner in all planes of motion, which can be hindered when it feels stiff and tight. These three planes—the sagittal, frontal, and transverse—are positioned through the body at right angles and intersect in the center. *The sagittal plane* bisects the body into right and left sides that move the body in flexion and extension. Bending forward is an example of flexion, while bending backwards is an example of extension. *The frontal plane* bisects the body to create a front and back half. Movements include abduction and adduction, lateral flexion of the spine, and eversion and inversion of the foot and ankle complex. Examples of frontal plane movements include side lateral raises or side lunges. *The transverse plane* bisects the body to create both an upper and lower half. This includes internal rotation and external rotation of the limbs, right and left rotation for the head and trunk, and horizontal abduction and adduction of the limbs. Examples of transverse plane movements include cable truck rotations.

Athletes benefit from flexibility, when done correctly in a controlled manner, it improves their agility, coordination, and overall performance. Flexibility allows for more efficient movements and helps prevent overuse injuries associated with repetitive motions. Stretching increases blood flow to the muscles, which can improve circulation and nutrient delivery to tissues, helping result in faster recovery after exercises. Flexibility exercises, such as yoga and gentle stretching, can have a calming effect on the nervous system. This helps reduce stress levels and promotes relaxation and mental well-being which pairs well with your nighttime routine.

There is a cumulative effect to flexibility training which means you will need to be consistent in repeating your stretches to feel the progress. Proper technique is key, however, as stretching incorrectly can do more harm than good. Know that cold muscles still need to warm up before stretching. Consider starting with 5–10 minutes of walking or biking before your stretch routine. Remember that not everyone has the same flexibility, so before you start comparing yourself to the latest gymnast or yoga instructor try focusing on your symmetry. Work to have uniformity on each side of your body as you progress. Start with your major muscle groups: calves, thighs, quads, glutes, hips, lower back, neck, and shoulders and repeat as needed.

Body Composition

Body composition assesses the proportion of body weight that is fat vs. lean mass. Your body's fat mass ratio to fat-free mass is used to determine if you are at a healthy weight for your individual body. This is important because too much fat can be associated with heart disease and type 2 diabetes. Therefore, attaining and maintaining the right body composition for you is important and as you can probably guess this means you are striving to have a higher percentage of lean tissue and a lower percentage of body fat. Looking at your body composition paints a more complete picture of health and fitness because two people can weigh the same but have vastly different wellness and fitness needs. Additionally, individual goals and overall health play a role in determining what is considered a healthy or desirable body composition for each person. Measuring body composition does not mean stepping on a scale like we so often do, rather measuring your body composition means using bioelectrical impedance analysis (BIA), hydrostatic underwater weighing, dual-energy X-ray absorptiometry scans (DEXA), or a body fat percentage calculator. BIA works on the principle that various tissues in the body conduct electrical currents differently. BIA machines have electrodes that you stand on or hold. A small, harmless electrical current is sent though the body estimating body composition based on how long it takes for the electrical signal to pass through your body. The electrical signal flows easily through lean tissue, which contains a lot of water and electrolytes, but faces more resistance in fat tissue. During hydrostatic underwater weighing you are weighed while submerged underwater. Because fat is less dense than water and muscle is denser, this measures the total volume of your body and, by extension, your body density. By comparing your weight on land to your weight underwater, the medical professional can calculate your body density, and from there, estimate body fat percentage. DEXA scans are often considered the gold standard for body composition measurement. Originally developed to measure body density, DEXA scans can also assess body composition. When lying down on a table, a machine sends low energy X-rays through the body. Different tissues absorb the X-rays differently, providing a detailed breakdown of body mass, lean mass, and fat mass in different areas of the body. There are various formulas and methods used to calculate body fat percentage, often based on measurements of different parts of the body. These calculations use measurements such as waist circumference, hip circumference, neck circumference, height, weight, and sometimes age and gender. The result is an estimation rather than a direct measurement, and the accuracy can vary depending on the formula used. These methods all have different levels of accuracy, ease of use, and cost associated with them. For the most accurate and comprehensive results, a combination of methods or professional consultations is advisable. These are typically provided by certain medical facilities, imaging centers, and specialized clinics.

    Recognizing the dangers of excess body fat, particularly in the abdominal region, highlights the significance of weight management for overall well-being. Excessive body fat, especially around the abdominal area, is associated with an increased risk of chronic diseases such as heart disease, diabetes, and certain types of cancer, while also being closely linked to metabolic health. Carrying excess body weight can also put additional strain on joints, leading to issues such as arthritis. Maintaining a healthy body composition, on the other hand, can contribute to better joint health, overall increased energy levels, optimal blood sugar levels, lipid profiles, and blood pressure—these are important to everyone.

Athletes and fitness enthusiasts often focus on maintaining or increasing muscle mass since having adequate muscle is crucial for strength, endurance, and overall physical performance. For athletes participating in sports that require specific weight categories, maintaining an optimal body-fat percentage is important for achieving peak performance. The great thing about understanding body composition is that you gain more information than just monitoring overall body weight, as a number, measured in pounds on a scale. Now you can distinguish between fat loss and muscle gain, providing a more accurate assessment of your progress during weight-management efforts. Since muscle weighs more than fat, it is possible for you to change your body composition for the better but gain pounds on a scale. If you were only evaluating your progress by tracking pounds lost, you would miss the fact that you have lost fat and gained muscle, which is a positive result. This is why I encourage my clients to look at body composition when on a fitness or weight loss journey and get a bigger picture of what is happening in their transformation, rather than relying solely on weight. While analyzing body composition, you can also guide nutritional recommendations to help you understand your body's specific needs, especially in terms of protein intake to support muscle maintenance or growth.

The body fat percentage ranges shown in **Figure 6-2** below come from the American Council on Exercise (ACE).[16]

FIGURE 6-2: ACE Body Fat Percentage Norms for Men and Women

DESCRIPTION	WOMEN	MEN
Essential Fat	10–13%	2–5%
Athletes	14–20%	6–13%
Fitness	21–24%	14–17%
Acceptable	25–31%	18–24%
Obese	Over 32%	Over 25%

---

[16] American Council of Exercise. Percent body fat calculator: skin fold method. 2017. Cited from the Centers for Disease Control and Prevention – National Center for Injury Prevention and Control. www.cdc.gov/steadi/pdf/STEADI-Assessment-30sec-508.pdf

The waist-to-hip ratio (WHR) is a measure that compares the circumference of the waist to that of the hips. This is calculated by dividing the waist circumference by the hip circumference. It is often used to assess body composition and health. The overall distribution of body fat is an important factor in health. Individuals with more fat around the abdominal area, aka having a high-waist circumference or an apple-shaped body, may be at a higher risk of certain health issues compared to those with fat distributed more around the hips and thighs known as a pear-shaped body. According to the World Health Organization, a moderate WHR is 0.9 or less in men and 0.85 or less in women.[17] In both men and women, a WHR of 1.0 or higher increases the risk of heart disease and other conditions that are linked to being overweight.

Carrying excess weight around the waist is associated with an increased risk of cardiovascular disease, type 2 diabetes, and metabolic syndrome. Fat around the abdominal area, particularly visceral fat, is also metabolically active and may be more closely linked to hormonal changes that can impact health.

You can determine your WHR on your own. Stand up straight and breathe out. Use a tape measure to check the distance around the smallest part of your waist, just above your belly button. The tape measure should rest gently on your skin, and not be pulled tightly. This is your waist circumference measured in inches. Then stand with your feet directly beneath your hips, measure the distance around the largest part of your hips, the widest part of your buttocks. This is your hip circumference. Now calculate your WHR by dividing your waist circumference by your hip circumference. It is important to note that while the hip-to-waist ratio can be a useful screening tool, it is not a standalone measure of health. Other factors, such as overall lifestyle, diet, and physical activity, also play significant roles in determining overall well-being.

---

[17] 2011. Waist Circumference and Waist–Hip Ratio: Report of a WHO Expert Consultation Geneva, 8–11 December 2008. WHO Library Cataloguing-in-Publication Data Waist circumference and waist–hip ratio: report of a WHO expert consultation, Geneva, 8–11 December 2008. 1.Body mass index. 2.Body constitution. 3.Body composition. 4.Obesity. I.World Health Organization. ISBN 978 92 4 150149 1 (NLM classification: QU 100).

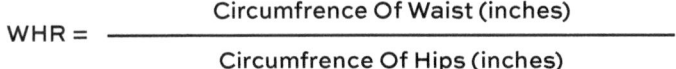

$$WHR = \frac{\text{Circumfrence Of Waist (inches)}}{\text{Circumfrence Of Hips (inches)}}$$

Record and track your measurements regularly using **Worksheet Q: Record Your Waist-to-Hip Ratio** to monitor progress, identify trends, and make informed adjustments to your goals and strategies.

ADDITIONAL AREAS OF FOCUS

In addition to the five elements of a fitness evaluation, I encourage my clients to focus on the following components in their routines and daily lives.

Balance and Stability

Many of us take balance for granted, but everyone can benefit from improving it. Balance is the ability to maintain an upright position and stay aligned with gravity. This includes coordinating the movements of the body's muscles, bones, and sensory systems as it involves integration of sensory information from the visual, vestibular (inner ear), and proprioceptive (body awareness) systems. Training and improving balance enhances neuromuscular coordination, leading to better control of movements—critical in many daily activities such as standing, walking, reaching, lifting, and running. These fundamental functional movements are essential for independent living and maintaining a healthy, active lifestyle. Stability refers to the ability of the body to maintain control and resist external forces. This involves the muscles' ability to contract and control the joints' movements to prevent excessive motion. This is essential for maintaining proper body alignment and preventing injuries during activities. Good stability allows the body to react quickly and efficiently to changes in the environment, such as sudden changes in direction or unexpected obstacles. Good balance requires good stability, and good stability requires good balance. When the body is stable, it can control the movements needed to maintain balance. When the body is balanced, it is better able to detect and respond to changes in its stability, enabling it to adjust to various environments and activities. Balance and stability training can help anyone at any age. The list of benefits is extensive—creating muscular balance in the body teaches your body to use its core for stabilization. A strong core supports the spine and helps maintain stability during movements. This, in turn, reduces the risk of back pain and improves overall strength. Good balance helps prevent falls, especially in older adults which can lead to serious injuries and a decline in overall health. Athletes in various sports, such as gymnastics, yoga, and martial arts, rely heavily on balance and stability. These attributes contribute to better coordination, agility, and overall performance. Proper balance helps distribute body weight evenly across joints, reducing the risk of injuries and wear and tear on the joints. Ways to improve balance include:

- standing on one foot
- heel-to-toe walking
- using a stability ball
- pilates
- tai chi
- yoga
- regular resistance training

Balance training is often incorporated into rehabilitation programs for individuals recovering from injuries, especially those affecting the lower extremities. It can help prevent reinjury and improve overall functional capacity. As you can see, balance and stability are integral components of your overall health and well-being. They contribute to everyday activities, athletic performance, injury prevention, and the maintenance of independence, making them essential for individuals of all ages.

Evaluate yourself at home with the Sit-To-Stand Test (aka Siting-Rising Test). This test gauges your ability to stand up from a position seated on the floor without using your hands, forearms, elbows, knees, or other points of contact for support. You will be evaluating muscle strength, mobility, proprioception, balance, and coordination. There is no time limit to this test, the goal is to simply sit on the floor and get back up with as little additional support as possible. Start in a standing position. Next, sit down on the floor, crisscross applesauce. Try to avoid using your hands as you lower yourself. Now, stand back up without using your hands or knees for support. You can score yourself on a scale of 0–10, five points for lowering yourself and five points for standing back up. Subtract one point for each time you used a hand, forearm, knee, or side of your leg for assistance. Your goal is to achieve a score between eight and ten.

The 30 second Sit-to-Stand Test is a physical performance assessment used to identify strength, balance, and flexibility. This tool can be used to screen your risk of falling and can be used at home by any individual, especially the elderly. The test involves recording the number of times a person can stand up from a chair and sit back down within thirty seconds. Start by sitting in the middle of a chair that does not have arms. The height of the chair should be seventeen inches. Keep your back straight with your feet flat on the floor, approximately shoulder width apart. Now cross your arms at the wrists and hold them against your chest and stand up to a full standing position as many times as you can within a thirty second period. Your score is the total number of stands in that time limit. See **Figure 6-3** below for a list of scores by age group. A below average score indicates a risk for falls.

Turn to **Worksheet R: Record Your 30 Second Sit-to-Stand Test**. Record your current test score in the provided table and continue to use this table to track your future scores to monitor your progress over time.

Setting Non-Exercise Goals

Remember: movement is moving. It does not always have to fall into a traditional "exercise" category. Find ways to take the stairs instead of the

FIGURE 6-3: 30 Second Sit-to-Stand Test [18]

AGE	WOMEN	MEN
60–64	< 12	< 14
65–69	< 11	< 12
70–74	< 10	< 12
75–79	< 10	< 11
80–84	< 9	< 10
85–89	< 8	< 8
90–94	< 4	< 7

elevator at work, wash your car by hand instead of driving it through the carwash, walk to talk to a co-worker or neighbor instead of calling, texting, or emailing them, stand while you fold laundry or get a standing desk for work, play with your kids, take your dog for a walk, do yard work or clean the house, volunteer at the food pantry, plant and work in your garden, or park your car far from the front door of the restaurant or store. All these activities will keep you from being stagnant in your day.

Active Recovery

Staying active is a vital part of supporting overall well-being, but it is important to give your body time to rest and recover. Training harder, faster, and more often can increase your risk of burnout, injury, and overtraining. This overtraining can lead to fatigue (physically, mentally, and emotionally), disrupted sleep, hormonal imbalance, suppressed immune function, and more. Your body and mind need a chance to rest, and active recovery should be a staple in your fitness routine to keep you feeling your best. Active recovery includes slower- and lower-impact movements and exercises to recover from vigorous training. These activities help to maintain a steady flow of blood and oxygen to the muscles, which aids in the removal of metabolic products that accumulate during intense exercise, reducing muscle soreness and stiffness. It can also enhance the delivery of nutrients to the muscles, promoting faster repair and recovery while maintaining flexibility. Low-intensity activities can have a positive impact on mental well-being, allowing you to unwind, relax, and shift your focus away from the intensity of your primary workout. This mental break can contribute to overall stress reduction. Now you are better prepared mentally and physically for your next training session.

It is important to note that the intensity performed during active recovery should be low enough not to cause additional stress or fatigue but sufficient to keep the body moving and promote recovery. The specific

---

[18] Center for Disease Control and Prevention. National Center for Injury Prevention and Control. (2017). Sit to Stand Assessment. STEADI. www.cdc.gov/steadi/pdf/STEADI-assessment-30sec-508.pdf

approach to active recovery can vary depending on individual fitness levels, goals, and the nature of the primary exercise routine. Try keeping these moves at a 4–6 rate of perceived exertion on a scale of 1–10. How many active recovery days you need will differ for every individual. It will also depend on the volume and intensity of a person's training, but generally one recovery day after three workout days should give your body enough time to recover and repair. It is also important to listen to your body. If you keep showing up to your workouts tired and sore, then you may not be fully recovered. Find out what activities reinvigorate you. Try these active recovery ideas:

- Yoga
- Stretching
- Mobility exercises
- Low-impact/low-intensity cardio
- Foam rolling
- Meditation
- Breathwork

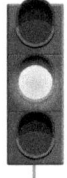

YELLOW LIGHT MOMENT

Turn to **Worksheet S**. It is time for your Yellow Light Moment. Ask yourself:

- How can I optimize my movement?
- What golden nuggets did I take away from this chapter?
- What can I start to implement immediately to improve the quality and quantity of my movement?

Write 3 action steps and start to implement at least 1 of them this week.

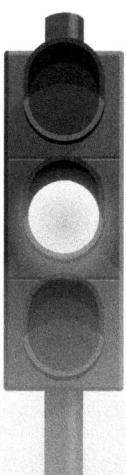

PART III
Empower

CHAPTER 7

The Power Of Commitment

WE ALL RECOGNIZE the importance of commitment, but do we truly understand its core? Commitment reflects an attitude of unwavering dedication toward a goal. It signifies a promise, a pledge, a contract—a deliberate decision to wholeheartedly pursue a purpose. Commitment is an agreement you make, serving as the base for all transformative changes in your life. In the context of this book, commitment involves taking clear steps and dedicating time and effort to nurture and boost your vitality. By focusing on maximizing your health and vitality, you establish the groundwork for a solid foundation, promoting structure and stability through firm decisions and consistent actions. When you prioritize your well-being, you invest in yourself. You actively choose to shape your life in alignment with your dreams, affirming self-belief, self-love, and self-respect by declaring, "I **am** worth the effort!"

The power of commitment lies in removing the words "I'll try" from your vocabulary and replacing them with "I will." When Yoda famously said, "No! Try not! Do or do not. There is no try," he emphasized that the first step to accomplishing anything is making a firm decision to act. At the beginning of this book, I asked you to adopt a simple yet powerful habit: asking yourself, "Does this choice support the lifestyle I am creating?" Not

"Does this choice support the lifestyle I am **trying** to create?" Speak as if it is already your reality. This is a lifestyle **I am creating**. Embrace it fully.

If you approach life with a "try" mindset, what happens when faced with challenges? "Do or do not" encapsulates the essence of commitment, urging you to make a choice, give your all, and stay dedicated. It suggests that your success is within your control. We don't merely "try;" we must commit wholeheartedly—mind, heart, and soul—to our ambitions.

Without belief in yourself and your objectives, it's easy to get derailed when life throws obstacles your way. Success often demands persistence, overcoming hurdles, and pushing through setbacks. Many begin with good intentions, but the moment results don't materialize quickly or as expected, they give up, make excuses, and miss out on the rewards of their efforts simply because they stopped. This is where commitment becomes crucial—it's the force that helps you endure challenges to reach your desired outcomes.

To achieve your goals, you must be fully vested. Step outside your comfort zone, embrace the challenges, and answer this call to action with resolute commitment and unwavering action toward your aspirations.

A distinction exists between simply "having an interest in" and "genuinely dedicating" yourself to your health and vitality. This difference is marked by the level of engagement, mindset, action, and perseverance you exhibit in upholding your well-being. Often, it's easy to settle for the bare minimum to stay safe, show a semblance of interest, and remain in familiar, comfortable territory. It's time to break free from the autopilot mode of doing the minimum required. It's time to embrace the next level of commitment and cease the self-sabotaging patterns in your life.

WHEN YOU ARE COMMITTED TO YOUR HEALTH AND VITALITY

You will notice these changes when you commit yourself to enriching your life, health, and vitality:

- **You have long-term focus:** Commitment implies a sustained, long-term dedication to your health priorities. This means understanding that health is not just a short-term goal but an

ongoing journey and that you will stick with it even after the initial excitement or motivation fades.
- **You strive for consistency:** Being committed involves consistent actions toward your well-being. This includes regular exercise, a balanced diet, sufficient sleep, self-care routines, and regular health checkups.
- **You are disciplined:** Commitment requires discipline of your thoughts and your actions. This means making choices that might not always be the easiest or most convenient, such as choosing a salad over a cheeseburger or going to the gym even when you don't feel like it.
- **You make a mindset shift:** Commitment often involves a shift in mindset from viewing health as an option to seeing it as a priority. This means making health-conscious decisions even when it requires extra effort or sacrifice.
- **You set goals:** Being committed means setting specific, achievable health goals. These could be related to weight loss, strength gain, endurance, flexibility, healthier dietary choices, sleep hygiene, stress-management techniques, or any other aspect of health you want to improve.
- **You take responsibility:** When you are committed you take full responsibility for your attitude and your actions. You acknowledge mistakes, learn from them, and make necessary adjustments.
- **You create healthy habits:** Commitment often involves creating healthy habits that become a natural part of your lifestyle. This might include meal prepping, scheduling regular exercise, hydrating yourself properly, practicing mindfulness, or going to bed at the same time every night.
- **You seek professional help:** When committed you are often more likely to seek guidance from healthcare professionals, such as doctors, nutritionists, personal trainers, or therapists, to optimize your health journey.

WHEN YOU ARE INTERESTED IN YOUR HEALTH AND VITALITY

Here are some things you will notice as your interest in your own health grows:

- **You show curiosity:** Being interested in your health implies a desire to learn more about it. You might read articles, watch videos, or listen to podcasts about various health topics.
- **You become more aware:** An interest in health often involves being aware of the importance of good health practices. This could include becoming mindful of the benefits of exercise, proper nutrition, sleep hygiene, and self-care.
- **You act occasionally:** You might take action toward better health, but it may not be as consistent or structured. For example, you occasionally go for a run, try a new healthy recipe every once in a while, or take a yoga class now and then.
- **You are less rigid:** Unlike commitment, being interested doesn't always require strict adherence to a regimen. It allows for flexibility and spontaneity with your health-related choices. Your health might be important to you, but it is not always your top priority so often gets pushed aside when something better comes along.
- **You have less-defined goals:** While your goals might still be present, they might not be as specific or structured as those of committed individuals. Your interests might fluctuate based on current trends, popular diets, how you feel that day, or exercise fads.

Both commitment and interest hold significance, depending on the context of your objectives. Recognizing this difference empowers you to make informed choices about where to direct your focus and efforts. Being interested allows you to explore new avenues and maintain a sense of curiosity. Yet, commitment is what cultivates enduring habits and routines, as you consistently invest time and effort in pursuing your goals. Remember, the level of success you achieve is directly linked to the investment you make in yourself, for life is essentially a culmination of your choices. Commitment demands intentional effort and steadfast dedication.

Failing to fully commit can result in stagnation, missed opportunities, and the squandering of valuable resources such as time, energy, and money.

Here are some steps you can take to commit to your goals:

- **Clearly define your objective.** Be specific about exactly what you want to achieve. Having a clear understanding of your commitment is essential to eliminate any confusion. The more detailed your goals are the easier it will be to create a plan to achieve them. The secret to having willpower is having "wantpower." When you are clear about what you want in life, it becomes easier to make decisions, stay motivated, and act in alignment with your goals.
- **Research and gather information.** If needed, gather information, resources, and knowledge related to your commitment. This could involve reading books, taking courses, talking to experts, or seeking advice from others who have succeeded in similar goals.
- **Set S.M.A.R.T. goals.** Goals are your road map to success. They give you a starting point and a destination to reach. They help trigger new behaviors, guide your focus, and help you sustain momentum as you have something concrete to commit to.

Let's dig into my top tips for writing effective, actionable goals.

Write SMART Goals

You can create **S.M.A.R.T.** goals by following the formula of **S**pecific, **M**easurable, **A**chievable, **R**elevant, and **T**ime-bound:

- **Specific:** Start by being overly detailed about what you want to accomplish and being able to quantify your goals. If anyone were to read your goals, they should be able to understand your exact end game without needing clarification. This is where the 5 Ws come into play. Ask yourself: **what, when, who, where,** and **why.** WHAT are you going to do? **When** are you going to do it? **Who** is going to be with you? **Where** is this going to happen? **Why** is this important to you?

The 6th W

I always like to add one element to the "Specific" part of SMART goals: **Write** it down. There is power in physically writing out your goals. Give yourself laser focus by writing your goals and looking at them every single day. Use an active voice and action verbs to state your goals. For example:

- I will run three miles every Monday, Wednesday, Friday, and Saturday at 8 a.m. with my friend, Traci, at the city park trail because it increases my energy to stay healthy for my family and helps me reach my long-term goal of 50+ miles a month, and 600+ miles a year.
- I will eat five servings of fruits and vegetables every day by adding spinach to my protein shake for breakfast, using peppers in my humus for my morning snack, having a salad with protein for lunch, grabbing a handful of berries and nuts for my afternoon snack, and steaming a veggie to add to my dinner plate. It helps me feel fuller, which keeps me from overeating and gaining those few extra pounds.
- I will limit my sugar to 30 grams a day by tracking my food and drinks in My Fitness Pal and cutting out the soda I would have as an afternoon pick-me-up at work. I will replace it with a glass of water or green tea to keep me from crashing a few hours later.
- I will meditate every morning when I wake up at 6 a.m. in my living room before I leave for work because it helps to focus my day.
- I will go to bed every night by 10 p.m. unless there is a special occasion. This will keep me feeling refreshed when I get up in the morning.

- **Measurable:** Your goals need to have a quantifiable objective so you can track your progress. This includes defining what data will be used to measure the goal and setting a method for collecting

that information. Examples include a journal, a checklist, a spreadsheet, or a tracking app.
- **Achievable:** Goals need to be realistic to maintain your enthusiasm in trying to achieve them. Of course, we want to dream big and shoot for the stars, but we also want to break them down into smaller bite-sized pieces. This is also a great time to learn something new to help you increase your chances of success, or to find someone or some resource that can help you.
- **Relevant:** Keep in mind that every action you take should move you closer to your goal. You want to make sure that all goals and subgoals make sense to the end game.
- **Time-bound:** Set a deadline and anchor your goals to a timeline. This is a great way to assess your progress. Create check-in points along the journey to make sure you are staying on track. Set a schedule to meet your deadlines and make sure you are giving yourself a realistic amount of time while also learning to adjust your process along the way.

Use **Worksheet T: Set Your Goals** to get you started in setting your S.M.A.R.T. goals.

Develop a Plan of Action

If you have big, long-term goals, break them down into smaller more manageable tasks and develop a plan of action. This makes the process less overwhelming and allows you to track your progress more easily. I love setting short-term goals thirty days at a time. When you set long-term goals, you can miss out on the urgency to get things done. It is too easy to procrastinate because you think you've got plenty of time—leading to missed opportunities, unreached goals, and unfulfilled potential. Instead focus on the next thirty days. Start by making an exhaustive list of everything you can think of that you need and can do to achieve your goals. Next, prioritize your list. Create a checklist organized by sequence and priority. Do not overload yourself with too many tasks in too little time. It is important to strategize your goals to prevent burnout. Add specific actions, deadlines, and milestones to each step on your list. Create urgency by asking yourself "what do I need to do to win **today**?" Remember, you will always find time for the things that are important to you, so start making your health goals part of your daily routine.

Make a Mind Map of Your Plan of Action

If I get stuck on where to start when setting new goals, I make a mind map of what I want to accomplish and what concrete steps I need to take. The main rule: don't overcomplicate or overthink this process. Begin in the middle of your paper and write down your goal. Now draw a circle around it. Next, without thinking too long or too hard start drawing lines out from the middle circle and list steps to achieve your goal. Add categories and sub-categories as you go, mapping everything out. Use the page freely, it does not have to be perfectly neat and tidy, which is the best part of this technique, you are just emptying your brain onto this piece of paper. Do not worry about putting things in the correct position, as you go on, patterns will begin to emerge, and sequential thoughts will become apparent. You can erase and adjust lines as you go. The most important thing is that if you have a thought in your mind related to your topic, be sure to write it down somewhere on the map. Every mind map is unique, but each one starts in the center, and radiates out like the branches of a tree. If you feel like you have more than one central topic on your mind, feel free to do more than one map! Check out **Figure 7-1** and **7-2** for example mind maps.

Allocate Resources and Identify Barriers

Identify the resources you'll need to support your commitment. This could include time, money, skills, tools, or support from others.

Brainstorm potential distractions, obstacles, or excuses that could hinder your goals. Take proactive steps to minimize or eliminate these challenges from your environment. Commitment will be the ingredient that helps you overcome obstacles. It helps you make choices based off your end game—not on what feels good at a given moment. It takes one good decision at a time repeated again and again to be successful.

Let's take a Yellow Light Moment and do a brainstorming exercise now to help you proactively eliminate barriers.

FIGURE 7-1: Sample Mind Map

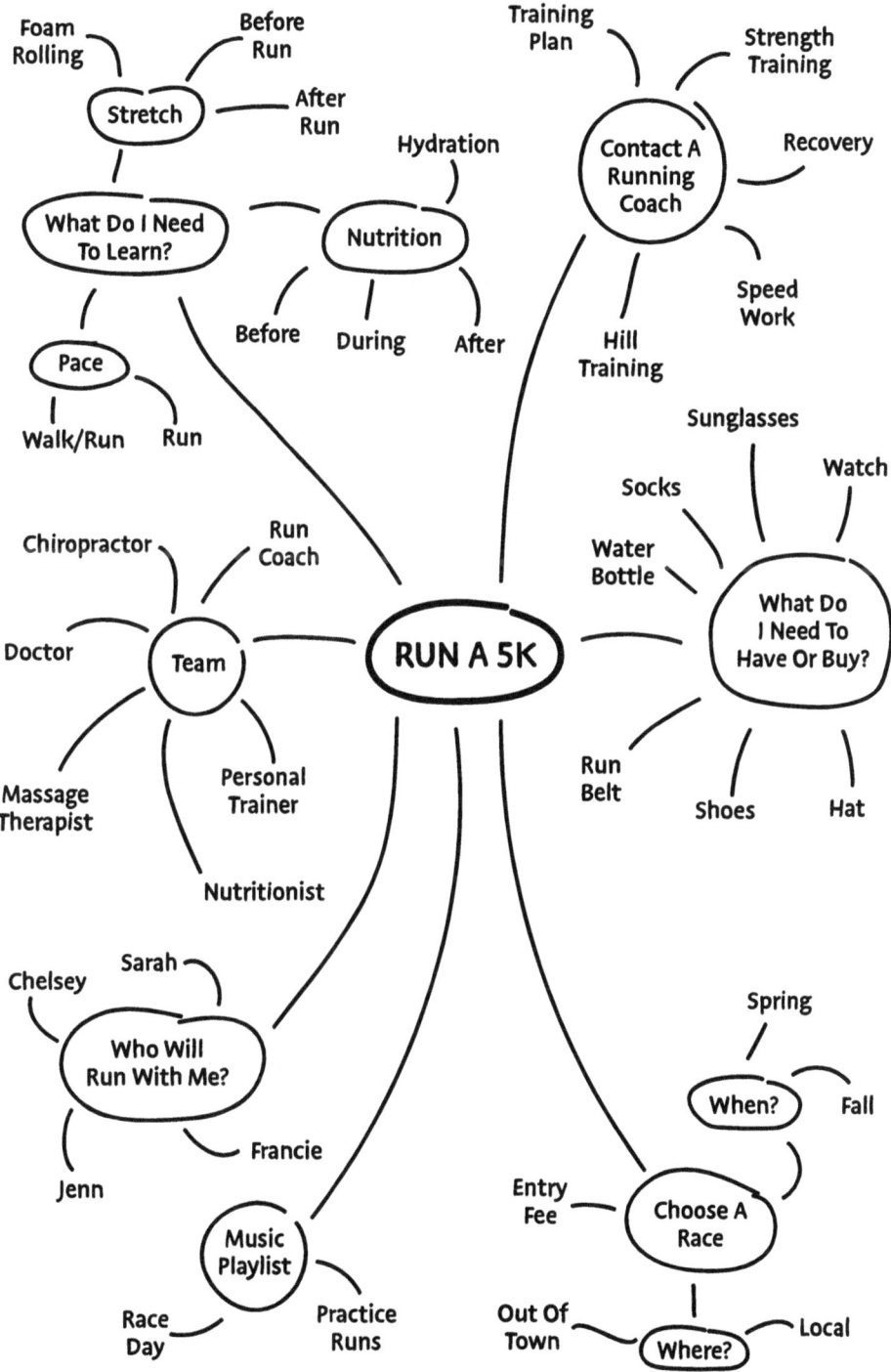

CHAPTER 7: THE POWER OF COMMITMENT

Start by identifying what keeps stumping you in your health and wellness journey. Is it being consistent with exercise, eating nutritious foods, getting enough sleep at night, or recharging your battery with some self-care? Do you hear yourself saying any of these common excuses or barriers for not prioritizing your health and wellness?

- "I have too much work to do." Many people sacrifice sleep to catch up on work or meet deadlines.
- "I can't fall asleep early." Difficulty falling asleep at an earlier hour can be a common excuse.
- "I'm too stressed to sleep." High stress levels can interfere with the ability to relax and fall asleep.
- "I get my best ideas at night." Some people claim their creativity peaks at night, leading to late nights.
- "I don't need much sleep." Belief that they can function well on minimal sleep.
- "I don't have time to cook." Busy schedules can make meal prep seem impossible.
- "Healthy food is too expensive." The perception that nutritious foods are cost prohibitive.
- "I don't know how to cook." Lack of cooking skills can be a barrier.
- "I crave junk food." Strong cravings for unhealthy foods can derail nutrition efforts.
- "I don't like healthy food." Preference for the taste of unhealthy foods over nutritious ones.
- "I don't have time to exercise." Busy lifestyles often leave little perceived time for physical activity.
- "I'm too tired after work." Fatigue after a long day can deter exercise.
- "I don't have a gym membership." Belief that a gym is necessary for effective exercise.
- "It's too cold/hot outside." Weather conditions can be a convenient excuse.

- "I don't know what exercises to do." Lack of knowledge about effective workouts.
- "I don't enjoy working out." Dislike for physical activity can be a significant barrier.
- "I feel guilty taking time for myself." Guilt of prioritizing personal time over other responsibilities.
- "I don't know how to relax." Difficulty in finding ways to unwind and practice self-care.
- "I have too many responsibilities." Family, work, or other obligations take precedence.
- "Self-care is indulgent." Viewing self-care as an unnecessary luxury rather than a necessity.
- "I can't afford self-care activities." Financial constraints limit access to self-care options.
- "I don't need self-care." Belief that they can function well without prioritizing personal well-being.
- "It's not a priority right now." Putting off self-care for a later time, which often never comes.

Take time to list every challenge and/or excuse in your health and wellness journey right now, being as specific as possible.

List every challenge in **Worksheet U: Mind Map Your Challenges** and be as specific as you can.

Now choose the **one** challenge or excuse you feel has the greatest impact on your health and wellness. Think of it as your greatest return on investment. This is the **one** area you feel, if improved would greatly enhance your vitality.

Next, outline every obstacle you can think of attached to this challenge. This is a list of every reason you feel you come up short from achieving your greatness. Do you feel this is due to time, money, energy, your work travel, no sitter for the kids, guilt of doing something for yourself, fussy eaters in your family, fighting insomnia, a chronic sickness, kids' activities, lack of knowledge, laziness? Think of every hurdle, no matter how small or how large you feel it is. There is power in writing it down and owning the reasons you feel you are failing. Be honest with yourself.

Now, brainstorm every solution you can think of for every obstacle and excuse you have just listed. Be creative and think outside of the box to consider every angle. Even if you think the solution is far-fetched and outside of your means, write it down. Ask others to help you brainstorm if you get stuck for ideas. Research solutions if you believe you have ideas outside of your wheelhouse.

Turn your solutions into small, manageable tasks. Now that you have concrete ideas on how to overcome your challenges and excuses let's put them into action. Start by picking 1–3 of those tasks that you feel the most confident with, to get the ball rolling. Yes, you can absolutely start with one. You are creating a to-do list. This is also a good time to ask others for help with this list if you think they can help you accomplish a specific task. Finding a **who** to help you with the **how** is a great technique when you know something might be outside your reach. This is also a great time-management tool.

Give yourself a deadline to start implementing the changes. Some of the best-laid plans are just actions on paper until you start crossing them off the list. Make that deadline **this week.** The idea is to start moving—no matter how slow, no matter how small—take a step in the right direction. There is no time like the present to get started on maximizing your health and vitality.

Build Accountability and Support

Declare and share your commitment with someone you trust and who can hold you accountable. This could be a friend, family member, mentor, or support group. Regular check-ins can help you stay on track. Surround yourself with people who will support and encourage you on your journey. Seek advice, motivation, and guidance from those who have your best interests at heart.

Hold Yourself Accountable

Do not procrastinate. Get moving immediately. You do not need to wait to learn everything about everything. Just get started. I was once told "ignorance on fire is better than knowledge on ice." You will learn as you go, so utilize the excitement of starting something new.

FIGURE 7-2: Eliminating Barriers Mind Map

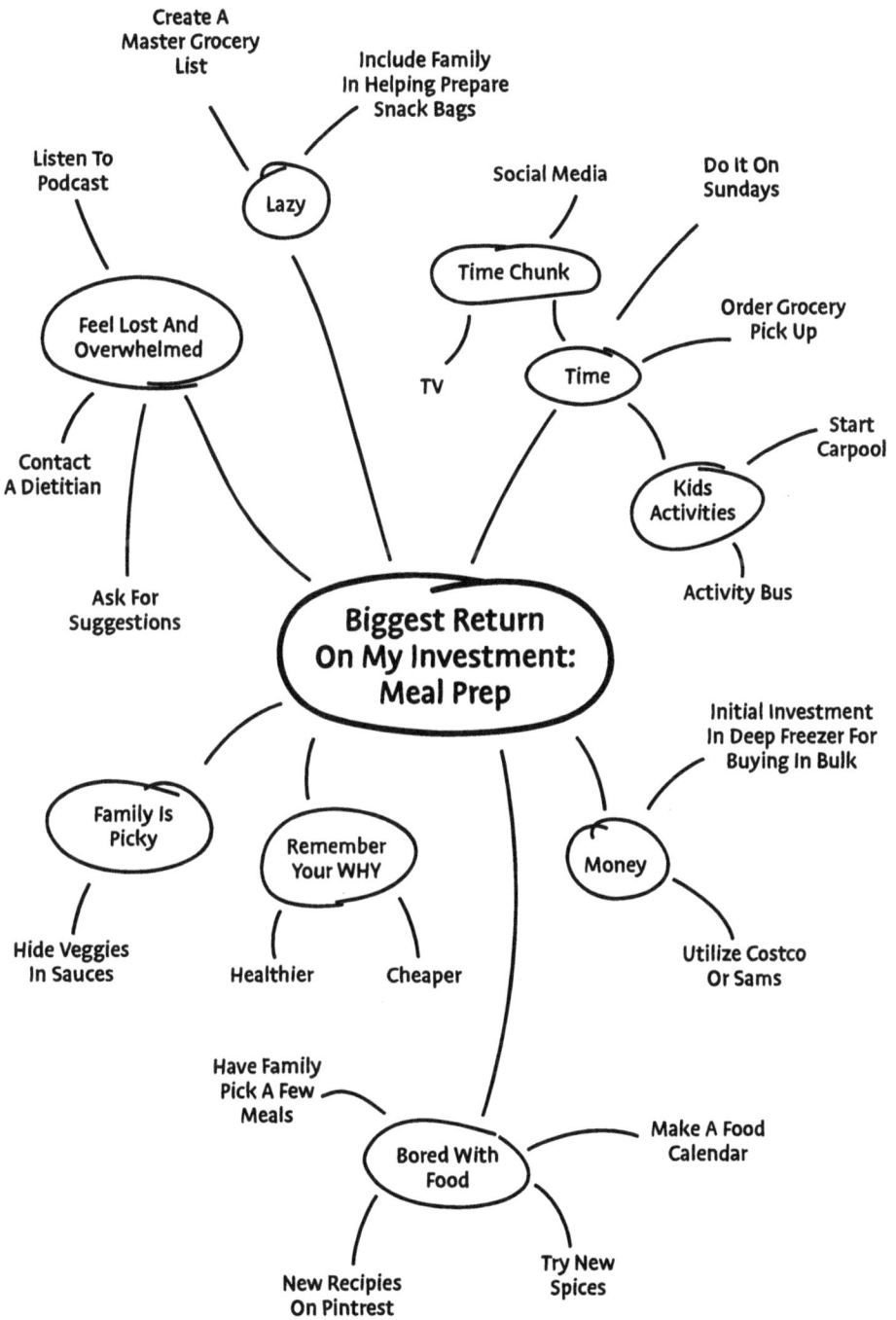

CHAPTER 7: THE POWER OF COMMITMENT   143

Do something every day. Look at your goals every single day. No excuses, every day, do something to move you toward your goals to develop momentum. Persevere through the thick and thin, the good days and bad days, getting hit and picking yourself up to learn from your mistakes. Develop determination and self-discipline. There is only one person who can stop you from succeeding and that is **you**. Assess where you feel you are "too busy." Are you doing the things that don't really matter to trick yourself into thinking you are being productive? Stop wasting time on lower-priority activities with lower significance. This includes activities such as checking email, posting on social media, reorganizing the linen closet, or any activity that is within your comfort zone.

Utilize reminders, visual prompts, or affirmations to stay focused on your commitment. This could be sticky notes, a vision board, or setting reminders on your phone.

Celebrate Achievements

Acknowledge and celebrate your successes along the way, whether they are small milestones or the triumph of the ultimate goal. I want to spend a little time here because I do not feel celebrating ourselves is given enough attention, and let's admit we do some awesome things on a regular basis. So why don't we recognize and celebrate them? Dedicating yourself to bettering yourself and achieving your goals should be celebrated no matter how big or how small. When you praise yourself for achieving your goals, you activate the reward center in your brain. This releases dopamine, a neurotransmitter made in your brain, which makes you feel good, and in turn makes you want to repeat what you just did. Dopamine is known as a "feel good" hormone giving you a sense of pleasure, while also giving you the motivation to do something because you are feeling that pleasure. Your brain is hard-wired to seek out behaviors that release dopamine in your reward system, so engage in activities that make you happy and celebrate your success! You are worth it!

Reflect and Learn

Regularly assess your progress and experience. What is working well? What could be improved? If necessary, adjust your action plan to stay on track.

This is a working goal. Know that you will continue to modify your tasks, obstacles, solutions, and deadlines as you learn what works and what does not. You can assess the effectiveness and efficiency of your plan over time and adjust it as your needs change.

Stay Positive and Persistent

Stay positive even when facing challenges. Persistence is the key to long-term commitment. Remember why you started in the first place and keep moving forward. Take time to visualize yourself achieving your goals. Imagine the feeling of accomplishments, the benefits, and the impact they will have on your life. One way to make sure you are staying positive is to look at your "I am..." statements. It is time to ask, "who do you say you are?" and fill your "I ams" with empowering and affirmative declarations: I am strong. I am confident. I am smart. I am healthy. I am vibrant. I am powerful. I am loved. I am worthy. I am dedicated. I am resilient. I am resourceful. I am relentless. I am deserving. I am committed. I am successful.

By following these steps, you can strengthen your commitment and your chances of success in achieving your goals and fulfilling your dreams. When you are ready, take a moment to complete the **My Commitment Page** on the next page to get started on setting your goals.

FIGURE 8-3: Sample Commitment Worksheet

MY COMMITMENT PAGE

I can and I will! I am worth it! I deserve it!

My goal is to:

_____
_____
_____
_____
_____
_____
_____

Because it will have the greatest positive impact on my health and wellness.

I will start:

_____
_____

By completing the following tasks:

_____
_____
_____
_____
_____
_____
_____

Signed: _____

Date: _____

Accountability: _____

CHAPTER 8

It Is *You* Against *You*

UP TO THIS POINT, you've examined the essence of your health and vitality and delved into the essential components of maximizing it focusing on your sleep, nutrition, self-care, and movement. You've also explored the facets of commitment. Now, it's time to consider the "who," the "why," and the "how." The "who" is a powerful way to define your aspirations, values, and the person you strive to become. The "why" involves examining the significance of achieving vitality in your life. The "how" will outline what sets this moment apart, enabling you to make the necessary changes to move from merely surviving to truly thriving. Keep in mind, *if nothing changes, nothing changes.* It's time to eliminate "I'll try" from your vocabulary and replace it with "I will." It's **go time**!

LESSON 1: DECIDE WHO YOU WANT TO BE

Have you ever taken the time to write a description of **who** you want to be? This can be a powerful tool for self-discovery and motivation. Your **who** is a statement defining your aspirations, values, and the person you strive to become. This involves introspection and reflection into your principles, beliefs, priorities, and joy.

To create a powerful and effective "Who You Want to Be" statement with a focus on health and vitality, follow these steps:

1. Identify key aspects of health and vitality.
   - Consider elements such as sleep, nutrition, self-care, and movement.
2. Reflect on your values and beliefs.
   - Think about why health and vitality are important to you. What motivates you to prioritize these areas?
3. Visualize your ideal healthy self.
   - Picture yourself at your healthiest. How do you look, feel, and behave? What habits and routines do you follow?
4. Write in the present tense.
   - Use present tense language to reinforce that you are already embodying these qualities.
5. Be specific and concise.
   - Clearly articulate the actions and habits you incorporate to maximize your health and vitality.
6. Include actionable steps.
   - Detail specific behaviors that support your health goals.

"I am a vibrant and energetic individual who prioritizes my health and well-being every day. I fuel my body with nutritious foods, staying hydrated and balanced in my dietary choices. I engage in regular physical activity, including strength training, cardio, and flexibility exercises, to keep my body strong and agile. I ensure I get 7-8 hours of quality sleep each night to rejuvenate and repair my body. I practice mindfulness and stress management techniques such as meditation and deep breathing to maintain my mental clarity and emotional balance. I listen to my body and give it the rest and care it needs, making self-care a non-negotiable part of my routine. By living with dedication, balance, and intention, I maximize my health and vitality, allowing me to lead a fulfilling and dynamic life." Visualize your **who** and let it serve as a daily reminder of your commitment to a healthier, more vibrant life. If you focus on this presence in your life with daily intention, your decisions and actions will align with **who** you are... even if you are still in the process of becoming that person. Who do you say you are? I challenge you to believe in yourself. Do not let anyone limit you, especially you. You are the one who decides. You are the one who commits. You are the one who acts. You are the one who chooses. You are the one who allows. You are the one who disciplines. Conquer you.

Let's utilize **Worksheet V: Who You Want to Be** to write your **who**.

LESSON 2: WHY IS IT IMPORTANT?

Let's go a step further to one of my favorite practices of defining your **why**. In the preceding chapters we have discussed why each of the four parts of maximizing your health and vitality is important for your mind, body, and soul. We have broken down how each of these points factor into your mental, physical, and emotional health and wellness, but WHY is that important to you? Going deeper than your health and well-being, why does it matter and what is **not** maximizing your health and vitality truly costing you? Your **why** is the driving force behind everything you do. It is your fundamental motivation. It clarifies your vision, defines your purpose, taps your reserves of energy, and sets your motivation into high gear. If it is compelling enough, your true **why** keeps you going when adversity strikes. It compels you to take risks, increases your courage and determination, and helps push you forward regardless of the odds or obstacles. Knowing your "why" enables better decision-making. It allows you to weigh your options against your ultimate goals and values, making it easier to choose the most aligned and beneficial course of action. It serves as a basis for accountability, a source to be evaluated against. Reflecting on your "why" allows for continuous improvement as it becomes easier to identify areas for enhancement and adjust optimized outcomes.

When trying to discover why being healthy is important to you, consider the following questions to uncover your motivations, values, and goals.

- What does "being healthy" mean to you?
- What are the specific benefits of being healthy that you value the most?
- What are the consequences of not prioritizing your health?
- How is neglecting your health impacting your quality of life, relationships, work, or long-term goals?

- What are your current health habits, and how do they align with your values?
- Is your health impacting your ability to travel and does that matter?
- What opportunities, experiences, or adventures become possible with optimal health?
- What emotions do you associate with being healthy (pride, joy, confidence, peace of mind)?
- What kind of legacy do you want to leave, in terms of health, for future generations?
- If time and money were no object, how would you be living your life and does your health affect that outcome?
- What brings you the most joy, makes you feel the most alive, and gets you the most fired up?
- What motivates you enough to get up early in the morning and stay up late at night?

Use **Worksheet W: Discover Your Why** to complete your **why**.

LESSON 3: WHAT GETS MEASURED GETS MANAGED

The essence of this statement is that quantifying and assessing various aspects of anything is essential for direction and improvement. If you do not measure something, can you truly manage it?

- You measure your life by years.
- You measure your health by weight on a scale or numbers from a medical report.
- You measure your sleep by the number of hours you rest in bed.
- You measure your food by calories consumed.
- You measure your stress by the number of hours you work in a day or how many meetings you have.

... Or do you?

Are you concerned, focused, and intentional about measuring the quality of life? If you were to do that, what would that look like? Do you **want** to increase your health span, not just your lifespan? If health span is defined as the quality of life, whereas lifespan is the quantity of years lived, how do you measure the quality of life so you can manage it?

I can say let's maximize your health and vitality by agreeing to sleep more, eat less, stress less, and move more, but what does that truly look like, and who is giving you the directions for that? When you measure something, you bring it into focus and make it visible. This visibility allows you to understand where you are, identify areas that need improvement, and track your progress over time. It creates a basis for performance accountability. You can analyze your trends, patterns, triggers, problems, and opportunities—your measurement establishes a feedback loop to adjust your strategies toward meeting your goals. Be inspired by this idea to be proactive in your health instead of waiting until the moment comes when you are reacting out of a state of desperation. By improving your sleep, nutrition, self-care, and movement you will increase your health span which will increase your lifespan.

Here are some ideas for measuring your health and wellness, allowing you to further manage it:

- Keep track of what time you go to bed and what time you wake up (trying to identify when you actually fall asleep is hard unless you wear a device such as a smart watch, Oura ring, Whoop, etc., but do your best).
- How many times do you wake up at night?
- Do you take a nap and if so, how long is your nap time?
- What does the scale say?
- Take measurements of your body (around your waist, hips, thighs, calves, biceps).
- What is your body composition?
- How many ounces of water are you drinking per day?
- How many calories are you consuming per day?
- How much sugar, salt, and fiber are you consuming per day?
- How much caffeine are you consuming per day?

- How many alcoholic drinks do you have per week?
- Do you complete more than 2.5 hours of moderate activity or 1.25 hours of vigorous activity in a week?
- How is your strength training progressing (how much you can push, pull, and hinge)?
- Do you complete 2 or more full body resistance training sessions per week?
- How many minutes are you meditating or spending in self-reflection per day?
- What is your blood pressure?
- How many servings of fruits and vegetables did you eat today?
- How do you feel after your meals?
- What is your waist-to-hip ratio?
- How are your cholesterol levels?
- What is your resting heart rate or VO$_2$max?
- How often do you connect with others via coffee dates, texts, phone calls, etc. to maintain a strong support system?

Turn to **Worksheet X: Measure So You Can Manage** to complete the worksheet on what you want to measure, allowing you to manage it effectively.

LESSON 4: CONTROL YOUR CONTROLLABLES

You are in control of two things in life: your attitude and your actions. This means you must be intentional and constantly ask yourself "Is this helping me become the '**who**' I am becoming?" It goes back to our original question: "Does this choice support the lifestyle I am creating?" Imagine if every thought and action you took aligned with this one question. Take time to identify:

- what or who is stopping you from doing the things you really want to do;
- what or who is stopping you from reaching your full potential;
- what or who is stopping you from achieving the success you want.

This might step on your toes a little, but this is the time to ask, "Are **you** the **who** in your own way?"

Learn how to distinguish what is controllable and what is a non-controllable; then take action to control those controllables.

THINGS OUT OF YOUR CONTROL
- The actions of others
- The future
- The past
- The opinions of others
- The outcome of your efforts
- Other people's boundaries
- What happens around you
- How others take care of themselves
- Timing

THINGS IN YOUR CONTROL
- Your thoughts
- Your actions
- Your attitude
- Your passion
- Your growth
- Your priorities
- Your choices
- How you speak to yourself
- How you spend your free time
- The goals you set
- How you handle challenges
- Your boundaries
- Your intentions

How powerful is that? You have command over your thoughts and your actions. Take charge of what you can influence, and then release the rest. That means you control being present in the moment, your words, your mindset, how you speak to yourself, what you give your energy to, how you use your free time, how you move on from failures, and the boundaries you establish. Remember we have already eliminated the phrase "I'll try." "I'll try" often serves as a pre-emptive explanation for potential failures, as if your effort is beyond your control. It is a way to excuse your possibility of failure or remove yourself from blame. You must accept 100 percent responsibility for the "Who" you are today. It is all up to **you**. You are in control of you. No longer create space for your own excuses, inner criticism, self-doubt, unhealthy habits, unrealistic expectations, people-pleasing tendencies, toxic comparisons, poor boundaries, energy drains, and lack of self-assurance. You might need to read that last sentence again. Let's get the work done on **Worksheet Y: Control Your Controllables.**

LESSON 5: NAVIGATE OR NEGOTIATE

You decide if you are going to navigate or negotiate the next twenty-four hours of your life. When you **navigate** your day, you plan it out like a road trip. You know where you are beginning and where you are going, having a definitive start and end point. You know the best road to take, what to pack, and when to take breaks; you plan for obstacles along the way and have made contingency plans if they happen to arise. You let others know where you are going and keep them updated on your journey. When you **negotiate** your day, you find excuses for why things did not happen. You talk yourself into believing it is okay to procrastinate or choose the fun and easy path instead of the hard and necessary one. You put your needs, goals, dreams, and beliefs on hold because they are not important enough to finish that day. There is power in **navigating** your day. I want you to attack every single day as if it were **game day**. Be pumped. Be ready. Give it your all. Keep your head in the day and stay focused. Work to make sure nothing derails you. I love the phrase, "You only live once. No, you only die once... you live every day!" Choose to live every day and to make the most of every opportunity to become better.

Take a few minutes every night to prepare for tomorrow; this is your navigation. Nothing is more stressful than being unprepared. Before you go to bed, make it part of your nightly routine to create a To-Do and a To-Don't list for the next day. What tasks need to be completed for yourself, family, work, and school? Do you need to pack your gym bag so you do not forget your shoes? Do you need to text a friend and confirm a lunch date? Do you need to prep your snacks and lunch, or set the crockpot for dinner? Do you need to download your next meditation or podcast to listen to on your commute? Also, set your To-Don't list so you do not exceed your ability to keep a life balance. You can even go a step further and time-chunk these items into your day. If you recall, time chunking is a technique in which you allocate blocks of time throughout your day to complete specific tasks. It allows you to focus on one project at a time instead of bouncing between different, smaller tasks. This increases your intentionality to get one thing crossed off your list. The next morning you will wake with a sense that you are in control which also sets a positive tone for your day. You now have the power to navigate the day on the path you have predesigned.

Use a planner to help you **Do The Dailies** such as the one below **Worksheet Z: Do the Dailies**.

FIGURE 8-1: Do The Dailies Example Worksheet

DO THE DAILIES

My goal to **thrive** today is: _____

_____

Sculpt It: Today's workout

1 hour is only 4% of your day!

Total steps/miles: _____

Ounces of water: _____

Fuel It: Today's Food

B:

S:

L:

S:

D:

Focus on your fork!

Reflect On It (exercise, nutrition, sleep, stress, water, energy, balance)

The good: _____

The bad: _____

The ugly: _____

Plan It and Work It (exercise, food plan, sleep/nap, relax/meditate, water)

Tomorrow's goal	Tomorrow's obstacle(s)	Ways to beat obstacle(s)

Regarding those obstacles... prepare to be derailed. It happens! Expect the unexpected! There is a project deadline that gets moved up, the babysitter calls in sick, you were not expecting to wake up with a migraine, the power goes out and you overslept. Take time to prepare for possible obstacles by thinking through the "if... then" of your day. *If* it rains in the morning, *then* I will hit the treadmill. *If* the babysitter calls in sick, *then* I will call my neighbor. *If* there is an accident on my way to work causing a backup in traffic, *then* I will listen to a podcast. *If* I forget to turn on the crockpot, *then* I will pick up a healthy meal from a restaurant. *If* I go to a social event after work, *then* I will drink two glasses of water before I arrive. *If* I am headed to a family Thanksgiving, *then* I will eat protein before I go and fill half my plate with veggies. *If* I do not get a good night's sleep, *then* I will have an active recovery day with restorative yoga and meditation. See how this works? You are preparing for the "what ifs" in life with your "if, then" statements. You pause. You course correct as necessary. You continue. If you are on a road trip you still must get to your destination. You do not turn around and go back home. You do not stop and say "Okay, I guess this is as far as we can get." You find a back road, a detour, another way around. It might not be the best, most effective route and it might take you longer to get there but, in the end, you still get there. One of my clients said it best: "There are more roads than roadblocks."

Be prepared to fail but fail forward. The problem with failures is that we see them as just that... failures. But failures are only failures if we let them defeat us. When we learn from them, they become part of our understanding, growth, and knowledge. Instead of perceiving failures, setbacks, and hurdles as something to be feared, we should use them to transform us. Remember you control how you react to failure. By shifting your perspective, you can now see those moments as chances for self-improvement and progression as you develop resilience allowing it to serve as a catalyst for your growth and progress. Failures may push you outside of your comfort zone, forcing you to develop new skills. If you stay the course, you can master these difficulties through your perseverance and determination.

I learned early on in my career that I was going to fail, but it was what I did with those failures that would define my success. Did I get hit and stay down or did I get up, learn from it, correct my course, and move on? You learn by doing. You learn by failing. You learn by never giving up. This is your growth process, and this is how you find success and what works for you. This is when you take a Yellow Light Moment. Examine it. Review it. Reflect on it. Learn from it. Bounce back from it.

Ask yourself three questions when you experience failure:

1. What went wrong?
2. What could you have done differently?
3. How can you improve next time?

Then challenge yourself to do three things:

1. Think positively
2. Be grateful
3. Keep moving

Flip to **Worksheet AA: Prepare Your If... Then Statements** and carefully fill it out. Completing this worksheet will help you clearly define your conditional action plans, enabling you to make decisive and effective choices in various situations.

LESSON 6: DECLARE YOUR NON-NEGOTIABLES

I find this exercise invaluable and one I feel worthy of repeating every quarter throughout the year. A non-negotiable, in its simplest form, is a way of setting your boundaries or your absolutes. A non-negotiable is an item that is not open for discussion, alteration, or compromise, but rather a declaration, an agreement, or a contract with yourself. Your list is completely personal, and you absolutely do not have to justify it to anyone because it is yours. In my personal life, my list consists of items such as, "I will never drive drunk or get into a car with a drunk driver. I will never start smoking. I will never intentionally pull an all-nighter. I will say, 'I love you' to my family every day." Now imagine the possibilities if you designed non-negotiables specifically related to the identity of your health and wellness:

- I will get a minimum of 7–9 hours of sleep every night.
- I will prepare my lunch every day and pack an appropriately portioned snack with the right amount of protein and fiber.
- I will drink half my weight in water (ounces) every day.
- I will complete thirty minutes of cardio 4–5 days a week and strength training 2–3 days a week.
- I will meditate for fifteen minutes every day.

Sometimes non-negotiables are forced into our lives. For example, you may discover a dairy allergy, making milk a non-negotiable item. Perhaps a diagnosis of heart disease or diabetes mandates a strict diet and exercise regimen for your long-term well-being. Today I challenge you to write out your non-negotiables for health and wellness, establishing your personal guidelines.

Turn to **Worksheet BB: Declare Your Non-Negotiables.**

LESSON 7: MAKING TIME VS. FINDING TIME

One of the most common reasons, complaints, and excuses I often hear from people struggling to find balance in their lives is **time**. "I just don't have the time to exercise. I can't spare the time to prepare meals or cook dinner at home. Finding time for personal self-care feels impossible. I can't manage eight hours of sleep because there's always too much to do before bed. If only there were more hours in the day." The issue with this longing is that time itself cannot be changed. Your day is filled with countless variables, but time remains constant. We all have the same twenty-four hours in a day. Therefore, it's not a matter of having enough time; it's about making enough time for what truly matters to us. Develop the discipline to establish clear priorities and then commit to them. Make a conscious and intentional choice to prioritize the most essential tasks that enhance your vitality, and then diligently work to accomplish them. Learning how to manage your time effectively is key to steering your life toward success.

It's time to change your perspective on time and reaffirm your commitment to balance your health and wellness by prioritizing the time for it.

Here are my top tips for time management:

FIGURE 8-2: Prioritizing Time

MAKING TIME	FINDING TIME
Intentionally setting time aside	Hoping there will be enough time
It is proactive	It is passive
Deliberate decision	Reactive response

- **Keep a time diary for one week.** This will illustrate the actual time spent on actions vs. the time spent thinking of or discussing an activity.
- **Make appointments with yourself.** Any activity that is important to you should have a time assigned to it. Schedule appointments with yourself to create time blocks for high-priority items. These appointments should have a start and end point and should be non-negotiable.
- **Schedule time for interruptions.** Plan time to be pulled away from what you are doing. Remember life is not perfect so you will need a margin of error in your day.
- **Allocate the final 15–30 minutes of each day to plan for the following day.** Consider this the navigation period. Don't conclude your day until you've completed this step. Sometimes, the most crucial part of your day is the time you set aside to organize your schedule.
- **Revisit your *why*.** When faced with the decision to make time in your day, remember **why** you are doing this and what goal(s) you are trying to achieve.
- **Let the world know you are busy.** When you are busy working on **you** it is okay to put up an *out of office* notice. In a world where chaos and overcommitment have become the norm, it is okay to establish boundaries between work and personal time—quiet the noise and focus on yourself.
- **Do not immediately give people your attention.** Practice not answering the phone, emails, or text messages the second you receive them. It is okay to disconnect and schedule a time to return all of your notifications.

- **Watch for time suckers.** There are many distractions that tend to send you down the rabbit hole. The next thing you know hours have passed and you have not accomplished anything except catching up on your streaming series, social media feeds, or the latest sports and fashion trends.
- **Get organized.** If it's going to the gym, then lay out your clothes before you go to bed or pack your gym bag. If it's meals for the week, then decide what you are cooking each night and write your grocery list. If it's getting to bed an hour earlier, then let your household know when you are retreating to your bedroom and set an alarm to turn off the TV and climb into bed. If it's meditating during your lunch break, then announce you will be out of the office or in a meeting during that time so no one can double-book you.

LESSON 8: BE CONSISTENT!

For any of this book to work you must do two things:

1. Find a system that works for you.
2. Embrace the suck.

There are numerous systems out there. Throughout this book I have incorporated a few tools for you to use, but ultimately you must find a system that works for you! This takes intentionality, energy, determination, perseverance, hard work, and consistency. The best piece of advice I can give you is to start small and simple. This is not "go big or go home." It is not "all in or not at all." Beginning with small steps creates momentum, starting with simplicity prevents feelings of being overwhelmed. Who hasn't said, "I want to lose weight, exercise more, eat healthier, sleep better, prioritize self-care, and reduce my stress level?" Yet often there is a gap between what we want to do and what we will do. We tend to set unrealistic expectations of ourselves. We do not surround ourselves with supportive positive groups of people, we fail, and we ultimately give up on ourselves. This time around let's be clear about what we want. We might encounter setbacks, perhaps even multiple times, allowing us to refine the system that works for us. Then we will repeat these simple and small steps daily... that is consistency! Remember that change and progress take time. Do not expect immediate results or instant success, it is human nature to resist change, especially when it comes in the form of challenges. That is why you must be resilient. This is when you learn, grow, and begin to thrive through your behaviors, thoughts, and actions.

No more complacency. It is time to change from who you have been to who you are capable of being. I want you to focus on one day at a time and I want you to **do the next 24 hours well**.

The concepts in this book are not in themselves complicated, but being consistent is hard. If you have a habit of quitting, it is time to break that habit. I can summarize what you need to do to maximize your health and vitality in one sentence; sleep more, eat nutritionally dense food in a mindful way that does not super exceed your portion limit for the day while cutting out sugar and ultra-processed foods, hydrate your body, prioritize self-care, and move intentionally every single day. It is the daily consistent application of those principles that make this a lifestyle in which you thrive—important, yet difficult. Doing it "sometimes" does not work. Doing it "part-time" does not work. Doing it "halfway" does not work. The key to success in any part of life is consistency. Stay focused. Find your rhythm. Give it your all. Keep moving forward. If you have chosen to do something, easy or hard, give it everything you have so you never have to wonder "could the outcome have been different?" There is no **what if** because you gave it all you could.

You need to create a system that you can follow, that is personalized to you, that you enjoy. Not having to think about it because it becomes who you are, is the game changer. These are your habits. By definition, habits are automatic behaviors we do daily. Habits allow us to work on autopilot. Some habits are positive and make us more efficient and effective, other habits can be negative, and are detrimental to our way of life. Once you have identified a habit you would like to change, you can work to swap it out with a positive or healthier alternative. Remember to think SWAP (Switch With A Positive). Start with one small and simple SWAP and then when you have found you are consistent with that one, add another and another. One at a time.

A practical method for developing a habit is to try habit stacking. Habit stacking is a technique for boosting productivity and changing behavior by incorporating a new habit into your established routine, pairing it with something you already do consistently. Begin by identifying a current habit that acts as your anchor or trigger. This could be something as simple as making your bed in the morning, brushing your teeth, or preparing a cup of coffee. Next, determine the new habit you wish to cultivate. For the purpose of this book, focus on healthy habits—remembering to take your vitamins, starting a daily stretching routine, or packing a nutritious snack for the day. Now, combine these habits by linking them together in your daily schedule. By associating the new habit with an existing one, you harness the power of routine, making it easier for the new behavior to become automatic.

OLD HABIT + NEW HABIT = HABIT STACKING
Make your bed + stretch for 15 minutes
Brush your teeth + take your vitamins
Prepare your morning cup of coffee + pack your snack for the day

To help create and track a new habit, follow the instructions for utilizing the two worksheets provided: **Worksheet CC: Habit Stacking** and **Worksheet DD: Habit Tracker.** By consistently using these two worksheets, you will be able to create a structured plan for developing your new habit and systematically track your progress, helping you stay motivated and on course.

People will start to see **who** you are as you have defined yourself. For example, my friends, family, and clients know that I do not go to the gym on Fridays because I work from home. I do not eat after 6 p.m. on weekdays. I always carry a water bottle with me. I run four days a week and strength train three days a week. I am learning to love yoga and found a way to make that a daily practice even though it is sometimes hard for me. They know I love to be outside and ask me to go for walks and hikes. I am in bed, without devices, by 8 p.m. on worknights. I open the gym daily at 5:15 a.m. with an energetic "Good morning, friends!" even if I have to fake it to make it on some mornings. It is my system, it is what I can be consistent with, it is who I am, and it is how I thrive in life. My goal for you is to write your own system so consistency is just a product for how your life works best for you.

EMBRACE THE SUCK

Notice I did say I have to fake it to make it on some mornings. Guess what? We do not always want to do what we know we must do, so we must learn to "embrace the suck." I first saw this phrase somewhere around mile twenty during my first Chicago Marathon in 2015. During that race, approximately 1.7 million spectators lined the streets of the Windy City. Many of these cheerleaders brought signs with them for the runners to view, and to add motivation to the runners who were drudging toward that infamous finish line. Among my favorites that year were: "Run faster.... The Kenyans are drinking your beer" and let's give credit where credit is due. That year the elite men's race was won by Kenyan Dickson Chumba in a time of 2:09:25 hours; and the women's race was won by another Kenyan, Florence Kiplagat in 2:23:33 hours. I was halfway through my marathon at that time. **Cheers!** "One day you won't be able to do this... today is not that day." **Amen, sister!!** "This is a lot of work for a free banana." I ate three that year and they were the best bananas I have ever tasted. "Smile! Remember you paid to do this." Yes, yes we did. But my absolute favorite sign was held up by a couple who knew that this was where many people hit the wall on their run and had to dig deep to finish the final 6.2 miles to the finish line. **"Embrace the suck!"** This sign stuck with me and became my mantra for the final miles as I kept repeating "Embrace the suck." The suck represented all the sweat, aches, exhaustion, and soreness I was already feeling. At this point of the run, it was all a mental game. There are two options at that point, finish or don't finish, and let's be honest—with only 6.2 miles to go **not** finishing was **never** an option. But I do have a love/hate relationship with this section of the marathon because you must dig deep and keep kicking your feet.

We all have moments in our lives when we must dig deep and embrace the suck. Whether it is an ongoing struggle to get your foot in the door of the gym to start exercising, the veggies and fruits you need to eat when the cookies and ice cream sound like a much better choice, the TV that needs to be turned off to go to sleep, closing your activity rings when a lazy day on the couch was the path of least resistance, or taking the time to be still and meditate when all you can think of is the next item on your to-do list. I am offering you my most motivating quote as a gift. To embrace the suck in your life right now. Dig deep. Keep kicking. And cross your finish line because you can do this, you are ambitious, and you are resilient! It is time for your Yellow Light Moment, and it is time for you to make the shift and embrace the suck so you can live your best life full of vitality.

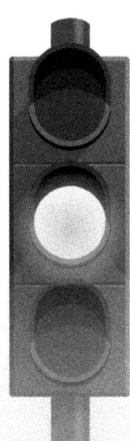

PART IV
Engage

CHAPTER 9

Proximity Is Power

WE KNOW social dynamics are powerful influences when it comes to behaviors. The individuals you choose to surround yourself with can significantly influence your thoughts, behaviors, and your overall outlook on life. Social groups, social pressure, and social media all help drive your thoughts and actions—both positively and negatively. Choose to surround yourself with positive people who not only inspire you but also challenge you. Seek out those who raise your standards. Intelligent minds that encourage continuous learning and curiosity. Connect with dreamers and visionaries who entertain your wildest ideas and always encourage you to chase your dreams. Engage with positive thinkers who view obstacles as opportunities. Spend time with people who make you laugh every day.

Collaborations are powerful, as we have the ability to elevate each other. I just told you to "embrace the suck" but that doesn't mean you have to do it alone. Build your dream team, where each person brings out the best in those around them. Just as hot coals stay hot together, individuals with similar traits, interests, and characteristics can come together to reinforce and amplify those qualities. People who share common goals and values tend to create a most powerful and impactful collective as likeminded individuals can maintain their enthusiasm, energy, and effectiveness when they collaborate. Surround yourself with people who challenge you, push you to be your best self, encourage your ideas, teach you, support you, motivate you, empower you, bring out the best in you, clap the loudest for you, and make you laugh every day. It is so much easier to create change when you spend time with people who align with your goals.

Find an accountability partner. Accountability partners are individuals or groups who work together to help each other stay focused, motivated, and on track to achieve their goals. The idea is to have someone who holds you accountable for your actions and progress. Start by having a thorough, open, and honest conversation with your accountability partner to discuss your progress, goals, challenges, and strategies. You should commit to regular check-in appointments and decide the time of day to connect, frequency of meetings, and a method for checking in (i.e., text, email, FaceTime, phone call, coffee date, walk, etc.). Regular and consistent communication is crucial for success, but it is also important to be flexible and adapt to changing circumstances. Accountability partners are part cheerleader and part coach and are there to provide honest and constructive feedback for you, helping to identify areas for improvement and celebrating your achievements. In addition to holding each other accountable, partners offer support and encouragement during both successes and setbacks. This positive reinforcement helps you to maintain your motivation. Having someone to share the journey with you can make the path to success more enjoyable and achievable.

At my gym, Vitality Fitness Studio, I offer accountability groups to support my clients. These groups take various forms: some meet 2–3 times a week for group workouts, others stay connected through texts as they participate in challenges like the 100 Miles in 1 Month Challenge. Some form teams to track their weekly miles on foot or bike, while others check in daily for a two-mile movement challenge. There are also groups dedicated to overcoming sugar addiction that meet weekly.

Our accountability groups are diverse, consisting of individuals of different ages, genders, occupations, body types, and fitness levels. Some members even reside in different states. However, they all share a common thread—they show up for each other. They exhibit consistency, providing motivation and support to one another. These groups serve as cheerleaders and pillars of support, embodying the essence of what it means to be part of a community focused on wellness and growth.

The incredible thing about today's technological landscape is the ease with which we can stay connected to others. There is immense power in surrounding yourself with individuals who uplift and support your decisions. Proximity holds influence, and forging positive connections can have a profound impact. These connections contribute to emotional well-being by offering support, understanding, and companionship. They provide a sense of security, guidance, and a platform for collaboration.

Here are some examples of associations and collaborations one can form to enhance their health and vitality:

- **Exercise Buddy System:** Partnering up with a friend, family member, or colleague to exercise together regularly, whether it's going for walks, attending fitness classes, or engaging in outdoor activities like hiking or cycling.
- **Healthy Eating Group:** Joining or creating a group of individuals who are interested in cooking and eating nutritious meals together, sharing recipes, meal prep tips, and hosting potluck dinners focused on healthy, wholesome foods.
- **Wellness Workshops:** Collaborating with local health professionals or wellness experts to organize workshops or seminars on topics such as stress management, mindfulness, yoga, or nutrition education within your community.
- **Accountability Challenges:** Participating in accountability challenges with friends or online communities, where members set specific health goals (e.g., drinking more water, getting enough sleep) and support each other in tracking progress and staying motivated.
- **Fitness Classes or Clubs:** Joining fitness classes or clubs tailored to specific interests or activities, such as running groups, dance classes, martial arts clubs, or team sports leagues, where you can meet like-minded individuals and stay active together.
- **Support Groups:** Joining support groups or online forums focused on particular health conditions or lifestyle changes,

providing a platform for sharing experiences, seeking advice, and offering encouragement to others facing similar challenges.
- **Mindfulness or Meditation Groups:** Connecting with mindfulness or meditation groups to practice techniques for stress reduction, relaxation, and mental well-being in a supportive and communal setting.
- **Community Gardens:** Participating in community gardening initiatives to cultivate fresh produce, learn about sustainable agriculture practices, and foster connections with fellow gardeners while promoting healthy eating habits.
- **Corporate Wellness Programs:** Engaging with workplace wellness programs or forming wellness committees within organizations to promote health initiatives, such as lunchtime fitness classes, walking meetings, or health challenges among employees.
- **Outdoor Recreation Groups:** Joining outdoor recreation clubs or meetup groups focused on activities like hiking, kayaking, rock climbing, or nature walks, providing opportunities to stay active outdoors while socializing with others who share a passion for adventure and exploration.

Positive connections often spark the exchange of diverse ideas and perspectives, fueling creativity and unique insights. They can also serve as catalysts for personal growth, as we learn from others and draw inspiration from their achievements. With this in mind, I extend an invitation to each of you to join the Vitality Community. Here, a group of individuals, much like yourself, are dedicated to thriving on their health and wellness journeys. The best part? You don't have to be local to be a part of it. Simply follow Vitality Fitness Studio on social media or join as a Virtual Vitality Client, and together, we can keep the fire burning. With Vitality, you will find motivation and accountability on your path. Stay **engaged!** Stay **encouraged!**

Use **Worksheet EE: Identify Your Associations and Collaborations**.

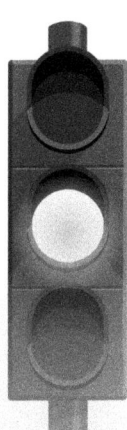

PART V
Ending

CHAPTER 10

My Final Thoughts

TWELVE MONTHS after I hit my second wall, landing me in the hospital, life threw us a curve ball. Our son was diagnosed with a bicuspid aortic valve at the age of eighteen. What started as Brian's chest pains turned into the in-and-out routine of multiple doctors, multiple tests, and multiple hospital visits. I first knew something was wrong when Brian walked out of the cardiac stress testing lab in one of St. Louis' top cardiology hospitals without having completed all the tests he went in for that day. Why would a cardiac hospital send him home and tell me to wait for the cardiologist to call, if there was not something wrong? Something in his echocardiogram was not routine. I remember going home and sitting in my office waiting for the cardiologist to call me with his results. Hours passed, which felt like days, as everyone knows who has ever waited to receive medical results. My phone rang shortly after 5 p.m. It was the cardiologist. I went into information retrieval mode while listening to the doctor's words. I had one job at that time—writing down every word he was saying so I could relate it to Brian, his dad, his sisters, and the rest of my family. I was also trying to think on my toes as to what questions I should ask him. When you have **the doctor** on the phone, you want to ask everything you can, when you can. After the doctor finished explaining what the tests diagnosed, I asked the question: "How do we fix this?" His words were few... "Open heart surgery."

The hours that followed that phone call were mixed with information processing, feelings of anxiety, stress, and fear... all regarding the unknown, but ultimately, I kept uncharacteristically calm. I did not panic. I did not cry. I did not feel nauseous. I digested the news and explained to Brian that the cardiologist wanted him to stop all activities immediately unless it was a "daily living activity." This meant no more sports, gym, work, or anything that would raise his heart rate, until they could do further testing to determine the extent of the damage.

Hearing your child's medical update and seeing him scared, sad, and anxious when you truly have no additional answers is a sobering experience. I could only comfort, listen, and pray. It became a waiting game... this was my wall of all walls, but this time it was different because I was ready. No one is ever truly ready to hear that their child has an 80 percent chance of having open heart surgery. No one is ever ready for the fear, worry, doubt, and anxiety that comes with that moment. No one is ever ready to take their twenty-year-old and fourteen-year-old daughters, Julia and Jessica, through the same cardiac testing to see if they too were born with the same congenital heart defect that affected their brother. The Bible verse that became our foundation was "The giant in front of you, is never bigger than the God inside of you." 1 John 4:4. However, because of our faith and the steps I had taken earlier that year to balance my life—I was hit, but I was not knocked down. I had the necessary strength for my family, and my body did not fail me. For eight weeks we walked in and out of doctors' appointments and hospitals. We had chaos in our lives, but we also had balance and peace. We continued to pray together. I continued to work out. I continued to work my "new" normal hours having cut back from the previous year when I was in the hospital dealing with my own health issues. I continued to meditate, practice my yoga, run my miles, program for my clients, run the business—and I continued to thrive. I was not already working with an energy deficit because I had made the choice to change the parameters of my life. I was navigating instead of negotiating. I knew what I was in control of, and I was controlling those variables. I had already committed to a change. It is about balance. It is about thriving. And it is knowing life is going to hit you with chaos and noise—but if you prepare for it, you will be ready for it.

Four months have passed since Brian's diagnosis, and I am finishing my concluding thoughts on this book. As I write this closing, I am looking out of a window from a cabin in the woods. It is winter. Christmas has just passed, and the New Year is a few days away. The trees are bare. The air is crisp. The sky is a beautiful deep blue with snow clouds drifting above. There is not a sound outside except from the rustling of the fallen leaves blanketing the earth's floor. In the past four days I have hiked in the stillness amongst the trees. I have prayed in the quiet peacefulness of the bright stars. I have stretched on a yoga mat in the great room in front of the stone fireplace. I have let the golden sun warm my face against the winter chill in the air. I have walked miles in the forest as snowflakes fell landing on my cheeks. I have gotten lost watching the flames dance in the fire as I listened to its crackling fill the empty space around me. I have watched deer walk by. I have photographed the reflection of this season in still waters. I have balanced rocks on top of each other in streams where my hands went numb from the icy water. I have watched the full moon peek in and out of the snow clouds drifting high in the night sky. I have slowed down to savor every bite on this trip, especially the leftover Christmas cherry cheesecake!

What is different this time? My life, my responsibilities, my health, my work hours, my stress level, my push, my sleep, my food, my energy levels, my exercise, my mental health... everything is different from that day on the beach in Florida. I am eating anti-inflammatory, whole, phytonutrient-rich foods. I am taking my daily vitamins and minerals. I am exercising. I am getting optimal sleep. I have incorporated deep restorative practices like meditation, yoga, gratitude journaling, breath work, and prayer. I have connected with friends and family, and I am living a life of meaning and purpose. I have shifted my perspective. I continue to manipulate the variables in my life and reevaluate what I am doing and ask myself if it is serving me on a monthly, quarterly, and yearly basis. This allows me to assess if I am surviving or thriving. My resources are no longer depleted because I changed the pace I set for myself—making it sustainable. Now I know how to quietly sit in the woods by myself and just be still. Now I know how **not** to burn the candle at both ends. Sitting still, relaxing, alone, with no work, no calls, no schedule, no texts, no commute, no lists, no expectations, no programming, no chores, no parenting, no grocery shopping, no cleaning, no bill paying, no emails... this is comfortable for me. And yes, I took time for another **Yellow Light Moment** as we get ready to kick off another year. This is Vitality Living!

Worksheet FF: The Vitality Scorecard is a powerful yet simple tool designed to help you continually assess and nurture your health and vitality. By taking a "Yellow Light Moment," you'll reflect on your habits in all four essential areas—Sleep, Nutrition, Self-Care, and Movement—gaining a clear snapshot of your current well-being. This tool isn't just for one-time use; it's a dynamic resource you can revisit regularly, whether weekly or monthly, to track your progress and stay aligned with your health goals. Each time you use The Vitality Scorecard, you'll uncover your strengths, identify areas for growth, and be reminded that vitality is a journey of small, intentional steps—not perfection. With consistent use, The Vitality Scorecard becomes your personal check-in guide, supporting your commitment to a vibrant and thriving life.

Use **Worksheet GG: Three-Month Refresher** to continue to take Yellow Light Moments to reassess your progress three months after setting goals. This allows you to evaluate your achievements, identify areas of improvement, and adjust your strategies or priorities accordingly. It provides an opportunity for reflection, adaptation, and maintaining momentum towards your long-term objectives, ensuring that you stay focused and accountable on your journey to success.

EPILOGUE

A New Motto

IN 2015 MY MOTTO WAS "EMBRACE THE SUCK." This year my motto is **"grit, grace, and gratitude."** These three words symbolize incredible pillars of strength to navigate life. I aspire to instill these values in my children as they journey through life. This motto is dedicated to them, embodying all my prayers and hopes for their growth into remarkable adults.

- **Grit** to seize every opportunity. To possess the passion, courage, determination, and tenacity to make daily changes needed to maximize their health and vitality and live the lives of their dreams.
- **Grace** to remember the saving, healing, life-changing power of God's love and to approach each day with a positive outlook, demonstrating resilience, understanding, kindness, and compassion toward themselves and everyone they meet.
- **Gratitude** to reflect on the positives in their lives, appreciating and celebrating the good, finding joy in the small everyday moments, and always making time for the people, places, and things that bring smiles, laughter, and happiness.

ABOUT THE AUTHOR

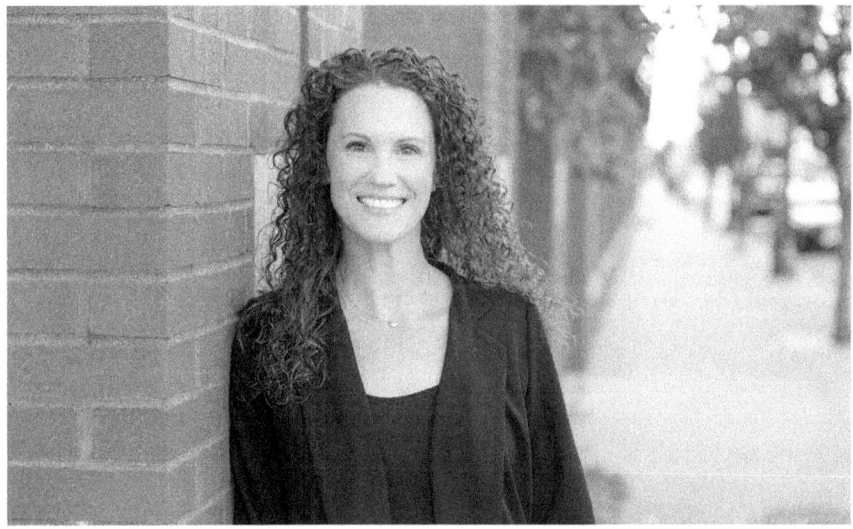

JENNIE PHILLIPS is a multifaceted fitness professional and educator dedicated to empowering individuals to lead healthier and more fulfilling lives. With certifications as a Certified Personal Trainer and Nutritionist from the National Academy of Sports Medicine, Jennie specializes in Corrective Exercise, Fitness Nutrition, Weight Loss, and Behavior Change. Additionally, she is recognized as an RRCA (Road Runners Club of America) Certified Run Coach, a Certified Stretch and Flexibility Coach, and a Performance and Functional Movement Specialist.

Jennie's diverse career journey began as a Biology and Chemistry teacher at Neuqua Valley High School in Naperville, Illinois, following the completion of her bachelor's degree at North Central College. Inspired by her passion for innovative teaching methods and outdoor education, she pursued a master's degree in curriculum and instruction with a specialization in outdoor teacher education from Northern Illinois University. Jennie's dedication to education extended beyond the classroom as she also authored curricula for school districts and state parks, exploring new avenues to engage and inspire.

A lifelong learner and avid traveler, Jennie embraces every opportunity to share her knowledge and insights in various settings, from classrooms and district institutes to corporate environments. She is passionate about educating individuals on achieving energy and vitality in their lives.

As the owner of Vitality Fitness Studio in Troy, Illinois, Jennie focuses on developing personalized training programs that blend therapeutic and performance-based fitness strategies. She is committed to empowering her clients to make informed choices and cultivate lasting positive changes in their lives.

Outside of her professional pursuits, Jennie finds joy in running, hiking, reading, and capturing the beauty of the world through photography. However, her greatest source of happiness comes from spending quality time with her family, exploring new destinations, and cherishing the blessings of faith and the grace of God in her everyday life. Jennie considers her family to be her greatest treasure and derives strength and inspiration from their love and support.

To contact Jennie, visit **www.jenniephillipscoaching.com.**

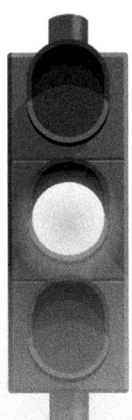

PART VI

Execute

YOUR YELLOW LIGHT MOMENT WORKBOOK

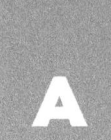 # Your Golden Nuggets

Golden Nuggets are valuable insights or discoveries you've extracted. These can be "aha" moments, lessons learned, or key takeaways. Use this worksheet to jot down your Golden Nuggets as your journey through this book.

A

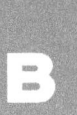

The Vitality Self-Evaluation

It is time for you to enter into a time of self-reflection. Start by finding a quiet space away from distractions, turning off your phone or anything that can disturb you. The goal is to connect with yourself to get an honest reading of how your life is going. Try not to be too harsh with yourself but look for truth in your answers. Remember, no one is the picture of perfection, so don't look for that. Let curiosity be your guide as you allow yourself to dive further into the reasons behind your answers. Consider whether there is a feeling, thought, memory, or belief connected to your answer. Write your answers down to better help you explore your thoughts and feelings. This is a great way to see if there are any patterns or triggers that follow your thoughts and actions.

Sleep

1. How many hours of sleep do I typically get each night? Am I consistently achieving the recommended 7–9 hours of sleep every night for adults?

   _____
   _____
   _____

2. How alert do I typically feel during the day? Am I relying on caffeine to get me through my morning or afternoon slump, am I having trouble staying awake?

   _____
   _____
   _____

3. Is my bedroom set up as an inviting space to retreat, rest, and rejuvinate? Have I made efforts to create a relaxing bedtime routine?

   _____
   _____
   _____

4. Am I taking naps that are too long or too late in the day that could be affecting my sleep?

   _____
   _____
   _____

5. How many times do I wake up during the night, on average? Are these awakenings brief, or do I find it challenging to return to sleep?

_____
_____
_____

6. Do I wake up feeling refreshed and energized, or do I often feel fatigued?

_____
_____
_____

7. How long does it take me to fall asleep after getting into bed? Am I struggling to fall asleep, and if so, how often?

_____
_____
_____

8. Do I value sleep, or do I feel it is time wasted when I could be accomplishing things?

_____
_____
_____

9. Have I experienced any changes in physical health that may impact my sleep (chronic pain, respiratory issues, etc.)?

_____
_____
_____

10. How would I rate my sleep on a scale of 1–10?

_____
_____
_____

Nutrition

1. Am I feeding myself to fuel my body or am I eating because I am tired, stressed, emotional, bored, or attempting to numb a pain?

   _____
   _____
   _____

2. Is my kitchen organized, clean, and ready to receive and prepare food?

   _____
   _____
   _____

3. Do I have the time in my day and week to prep the food I need to support my work hours, family, exercise, and health issues?

   _____
   _____
   _____

4. If I do not have the time to prep and cook food, do I have a system set in place for quick on-the-go healthy, and delicious meals?

   _____
   _____
   _____

5. How many meals am I cooking at home that are fresh vs. what is prepackaged, ultra-processed, or fast food?

   _____
   _____
   _____

6. Is food bringing me joy or do I feel constant guilt and shame around eating?

   _____
   _____
   _____

7. Am I craving sweets, caffeine, salt, and carbs?

　_____
　_____
　_____

8. Am I constantly hungry, or do I wake up hungry in the middle of the night?

　_____
　_____
　_____

9. How much water do I drink during a typical day?

　_____
　_____
　_____

10. How would I rate the quality and quantity of my meals, snacks, and drinks on a scale of 1–10?

　_____
　_____
　_____

Self-Care

1. Do I know the difference between being tired because I need rest, or because I need peace?

　_____
　_____
　_____

2. Am I having mood swings, or do I lack the ability to deal with the day-to-day hurdles that come my way?

　_____
　_____
　_____

3. Am I feeling centered and nurturing my spiritual well-being and connection with my faith during challenging times?

___

4. Am I setting boundaries so I can take time to recharge myself?

___

5. Do I need a therapist to help me build tools and skills to weather the harder parts of life?

___

6. Am I prioritizing self-care, or do I feel guilty for taking a timeout or taking time away from my family, for myself?

___

7. Do I ever just sit quietly to be alone with my thoughts, or is every minute of my day already scheduled and full of noise?

___

8. Am I practicing stress-management techniques, such as deep breathing and meditation?

___

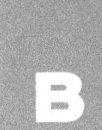

9. Do I maintain heathy relationships and connect regularly with supportive friends and family?

10. How would I rate my stress level on a scale of 1–10?

Movement

1. Am I incorporating 4–5 days of cardio and 2–3 days of strength training each week?

2. Am I completing intentional exercise during my day or am I counting my regular routine as an activity?

3. Do I find joy in exercising, or does it feel like an obligation?

4. Am I stretching as active recovery after my workouts?

5. Do I need to find ways to mix up my exercise routine (i.e., yoga, swimming, a group fitness class, hiking a new nature trail)?

_____
_____
_____

6. Do I feel confident knowing what I need to do to exercise my body, or do I need to hire a professional to get me started, vary my routines, and hold me accountable?

_____
_____
_____

7. Do I find excuses for why I cannot go to the gym or get regular exercise?

_____
_____

8. Do I find myself socializing at the gym instead of keeping myself accountable for why I am there?

_____
_____

9. Do I truly believe regular exercise is important to my health and should be made a priority?

_____
_____
_____

10. How would I rate my cardiorespiratory endurance, muscular strength, muscular endurance, flexibility, and body composition on a scale of 1–10?

_____
_____
_____

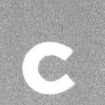 # Yellow Light Moment To Find Your Zzzs

How can I optimize my sleep routine?

_____
_____
_____
_____
_____
_____

What golden nuggets did I take away from this chapter?

_____
_____
_____
_____
_____
_____

What can I start to implement immediately to improve the quality and quantity of my sleep?

_____
_____
_____
_____

Write **3 action steps** and start to implement at least 1 of them this week.

1. _____
   _____
   _____

2. _____
   _____
   _____

3. _____
   _____
   _____

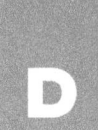 # Food Diary: Steps

Keeping a daily food diary can be an effective way to monitor your eating habits and help you reach your dietary goals. Here are some simple steps to get started:

1. Choose Your Diary Format
   - **Paper Journal:** Use a notebook or a specially designed food diary.
   - **Digital App:** Download a food tracking app on your smartphone.
   - **Spreadsheet:** Create a digital log using a program like Excel or Google Sheets.
2. Record Each Meal, Snack, and Drink
   - **What to Include:** Note the type of food and drink, portion sizes, and any added ingredients (e.g., dressings, sauces).
   - **Timing:** Write down the time of each meal or snack.
   - **Details Matter:** Be as specific as possible (e.g., 1 cup of cooked brown rice, 2 tablespoons of peanut butter).
3. Track Nutritional Information
   - **Calories:** If you're counting calories, include them for each item.
   - **Macros:** Track macronutrients (carbohydrates, proteins, fats) if relevant to your goals.
   - **Micros:** Note vitamins and minerals if you have specific nutritional targets.
4. Reflect on Your Eating Habits
   - **Hunger Levels:** Record how hungry you were before eating.
   - **Emotions:** Note any emotions you were feeling (e.g., stress, boredom) that may have influenced your eating.
   - **Environment:** Mention where you ate (e.g., at the table, in front of the TV) and who you were with.
5. Review Your Entries Daily
   - **Identify Patterns:** Look for trends in your eating habits, such as times of day when you tend to overeat or skip meals.
   - **Adjust as Needed:** Use your observations to make healthier choices, plan balanced meals, and control portion sizes.
6. Set Goals and Track Progress
   - **Short-term Goals:** Set daily or weekly goals, such as increasing vegetable intake or reducing sugary snacks.
   - **Long-term Goals:** Keep an eye on broader objectives, like weight loss, muscle gain, or improved energy levels.
   - **Monitor Changes:** Regularly compare your current entries with past logs to see your progress and adjust your strategies.

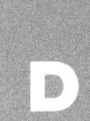

7. Stay Consistent
   - **Daily Entries:** Aim to log your food intake every day, even on weekends and holidays.
   - **Honesty is Key:** Be truthful in your recordings, as accuracy will help you achieve your goals.

By following these steps, you can effectively use a food diary to enhance your awareness of your eating habits and support your health and wellness goals.

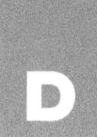# Food Diary: Worksheet

List what you ate and drank for breakfast, lunch, dinner, and snacks. Record the amounts and the calories of each item.

BREAKFAST

_____
_____
_____ Calories _____

LUNCH

_____
_____
_____ Calories _____

DINNER

_____
_____
_____ Calories: _____

SNACKS

_____
_____
_____ Calories _____

Glasses of water I drank today _____
My mood today _____ Total Calories _____

Notes_____
_____
_____
_____
_____
_____

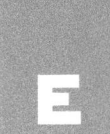 # Meal Planners: Steps

Using a monthly meal planner can help you stay organized, save time, and maintain a balanced diet. Here's how to get started:

1. Plan Your Meals in Advance
   - **Monthly Overview:** Look at the entire month to plan your meals, considering any special events, holidays, or busy days.
   - **Weekly Focus:** Break down the month into weeks for more detailed planning. Decide on breakfast, lunch, dinner, and snacks for each day.
2. Balance Your Meals
   - **Nutritional Goals:** Ensure each meal includes a balance of proteins, carbohydrates, fats, and plenty of fruits and vegetables.
   - **Variety:** Include a variety of foods to avoid monotony and ensure a range of nutrients.
3. Create a Master Shopping List
   - **Weekly Lists:** Based on your meal plan, create a shopping list for each week.
   - **Bulk Items:** Note items you can buy in bulk and use throughout the month.
4. Schedule Prep Days
   - **Batch Cooking:** Allocate specific days for meal prep, such as Sundays, to cook and portion meals for the upcoming week.
   - **Storage:** Plan for how you will store prepped meals (e.g., refrigerator, freezer).
5. Adjust as Needed
   - **Flexibility:** Be prepared to adjust if plans change or if you have leftovers.
   - **Feedback:** After each week, review what worked well and what didn't, and adjust future plans accordingly.

E Meal Planners: Monthly

WEEK 1

MON	
TUE	
WED	
THU	
FRI	
SAT	
SUN	

WEEK 2

MON	
TUE	
WED	
THU	
FRI	
SAT	
SUN	

WEEK 3

MON	
TUE	
WED	
THU	
FRI	
SAT	
SUN	

WEEK 4

MON	
TUE	
WED	
THU	
FRI	
SAT	
SUN	

Meal Planners: Weekly

	BREAKFAST	LUNCH	DINNER
MON			
TUE			
WED			
THU			
FRI			
SAT			
SUN			

THIS WEEK'S SNACKS

SHOPPING LIST

FAMILY SUGGESTIONS

F Grocery List Organizer

FRUITS	VEGGIES	MEATS

GRAINS	FREEZER	DAIRY

DELI	CONDIMENTS	CANNED GOODS

BEVERAGES	BAKERY	MISC

EXTRAS

Grocery Shopping Checklist

- **Check the Pantry and Fridge:** Before making your list, take inventory of what you already have. This prevents buying duplicates and ensures you use up ingredients on hand.
- **Plan Based on Recipes:** Use your meal plan to generate a comprehensive shopping list. List out all the ingredients needed for each recipe, including quantities.
- **Organize Your List:** Group items by categories (produce, dairy, meats, pantry staples) to make shopping more efficient. Consider using a grocery shopping app for ease of use and organization.

Grocery Shopping Checklist

1. FRESH PRODUCE
- ☐ Apples
- ☐ Bananas
- ☐ Oranges
- ☐ Spinach
- ☐ Broccoli
- ☐ Carrots
- ☐ Bell peppers
- ☐ Tomatoes
- ☐ Avocado

2. DAIRY AND EGGS
- ☐ Milk (or dairy-free alternative)
- ☐ Yogurt
- ☐ Cheese
- ☐ Eggs
- ☐ Butter (or dairy-free alternative)

3. PROTEIN
- ☐ Chicken breasts
- ☐ Lean ground turkey
- ☐ Salmon fillets
- ☐ Tofu (or other plant-based protein)
- ☐ Beans

4. GRAINS AND LEGUMES
- ☐ Whole wheat bread
- ☐ Brown rice
- ☐ Quinoa
- ☐ Oats
- ☐ Lentils

5. FROZEN FOODS
- ☐ Frozen berries
- ☐ Frozen vegetables
- ☐ Frozen shrimp
- ☐ Frozen edamame

6. PANTRY STAPLES
- ☐ Olive oil
- ☐ Vinegar (e.g., balsamic, apple cider)
- ☐ Spices
- ☐ Canned tomatoes
- ☐ Whole grain pasta
- ☐ Canned beans
- ☐ Nut butter (e.g., peanut butter, almond butter)
- ☐ Honey (or other sweeteners)

7. SNACKS AND TREATS
- ☐ Nuts
- ☐ Seeds
- ☐ Whole grain crackers
- ☐ Hummus
- ☐ Dark chocolate
- ☐ Popcorn
- ☐ Granola bars

8. BEVERAGES
- ☐ Water
- ☐ Herbal tea
- ☐ Coffee
- ☐ Sparkling water
- ☐ Juice

9. HOUSEHOLD ITEMS
- ☐ Paper towels
- ☐ Toilet paper
- ☐ Cleaning supplies
- ☐ Laundry detergent
- ☐ Dish soap

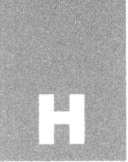

Yellow Light Moment To Focus On Your Fork

How can I optimize my nutrition?

_____
_____
_____
_____
_____

What golden nuggets did I take away from this chapter?

_____
_____
_____
_____
_____

What can I start to implement immediately to improve the quality and value of my food?

_____
_____
_____
_____

Write **3 action steps** and start to implement at least 1 of them this week.

1. _____
_____

2. _____
_____

3. _____
_____

Time Chunking Your Day

Time chunking is a productivity technique where you allocate specific blocks of time to focus on particular tasks or activities, enhancing efficiency and reducing distractions.

Example

NORMAL SCHEDULE

9:00	Emails
9:30	Social Media
10:00	Emails and Client Profiles
11:00	Meeting
12:00	Lunch
1:00	Create Client Profile
1:30	Emails
2:00	Meeting
3:00	Meeting
3:30	Client Profile
4:00	Meeting
5:00	Email

TIME CHUNK SCHEDULE

9:00–12:00
Create Client Profiles

12:00
Lunch

1:00–3:00
Emails and Messages

3:00–5:00
Meetings

5:00
Plan For Tomorrow

Block off your day in "chunks" by scheduling more than one hour at a time for your to-dos

5:00 _____
6:00 _____
7:00 _____
8:00 _____
9:00 _____
10:00 _____
11:00 _____
12:00 _____
1:00 _____
2:00 _____
3:00 _____
4:00 _____
5:00 _____
6:00 _____
7:00 _____
8:00 _____
9:00 _____
10:00 _____

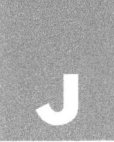

Yellow Light Moment Journal Page

Take a Yellow Light Moment to assess your health and vitality today. Think about your physical, emotional, and mental state. What positive actions or habits did you practice today that enhanced your health and wellness? Are there specific areas you feel could use more attention or improvement? Reflect on any obstacles you may be experiencing and how to overcome them. Share your reflections and observations here.

Date _____

Focus of My Day/Week _____

Reflections

_____
_____
_____
_____
_____
_____
_____
_____
_____
_____
_____
_____
_____
_____
_____
_____
_____
_____
_____

Rate Your Vitality Level: 1   2   3   4   5   6   7   8   9   10

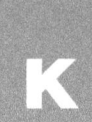

Blank Journal Page

Using a prompt from Chapter 5 or a topic of your own, use this space to journal today.

Date _____

Today's Journal Topic _____

_____
_____
_____
_____
_____
_____
_____
_____
_____
_____
_____
_____
_____
_____
_____
_____
_____
_____
_____
_____
_____
_____
_____
_____
_____
_____

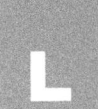

Writing Your Mantra

Write out your favorite mantra(s) from Chapter 5 or create one of your own.

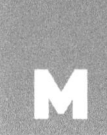 # Saying "No"

Enhancing your health and vitality involves making conscious decisions to let go of or say no to certain habits and commitments. Here's a guide to help you identify and articulate these changes in the areas of nutrition, movement, sleep, and self-care.

1. Find a Quiet Space
   - **Environment:** Choose a peaceful place where you can focus without distractions.
   - **Materials:** Have a notebook or digital device ready for writing.
2. Reflect on Each Area
   - **Sleep:** Reflect on your sleep quality, duration, and bedtime habits.
   - **Nutrition:** Consider your eating habits, food choices, and meal patterns.
   - **Self-Care:** Assess your self-care practices, stress management, and relaxation techniques.
   - **Movement:** Think about your physical activity levels and exercise routines.
3. Identify What to Let Go or Say No To
   - **Habits:** List specific habits that negatively impact your health in each area.
   - **Commitments:** Consider commitments that interfere with your ability to prioritize these aspects of your health.
4. Write Your List
   - **Be Specific:** Clearly state what you are willing to let go of or say no to in each area.
   - **Positive Framing:** Focus on the benefits you will gain by making these changes.
5. Create an Action Plan
   - **Steps:** Outline specific actions to let go of or say no to the identified habits and commitments.
   - **Timeline:** Set a realistic timeline for implementing these changes.
   - **Support:** Identify any support you may need (e.g., accountability partner, professional advice).
6. Review and Reflect
   - **Regular Check-Ins:** Schedule regular times to review your list and reflect on your progress.
   - **Adjust as Needed:** Be flexible and adjust as your priorities and circumstances evolve.

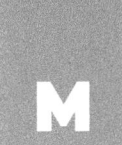

Example List

NUTRITION:
- **Let Go:** "I will let go of consuming sugary snacks after dinner."
- **Action Plan:** Replace sugary snacks with healthier options like fruit or nuts. Set a goal to implement this change over the next two weeks.
- **Say No To:** "I will say no to skipping meals due to a busy schedule."
- **Action Plan:** Plan and prepare balanced meals ahead of time to ensure I eat regularly. Start meal prepping on Sundays.

MOVEMENT:
- **Let Go:** "I will let go of using the elevator and start taking the stairs more often."
- **Action Plan:** Commit to taking the stairs at least once a day, gradually increasing frequency.
- **Say No To:** "I will say no to prolonged periods of sitting without breaks."
- **Action Plan:** Set a timer to remind me to stand and stretch every hour during work.

SLEEP:
- **Let Go:** "I will let go of using electronic devices an hour before bedtime."
- **Action Plan:** Establish a bedtime routine that includes reading a book or other relaxing activities instead of screen time.
- **Say No To:** "I will say no to late-night caffeine consumption."
- **Action Plan:** Switch to herbal tea or water after 6 p.m.

SELF-CARE:
- **Let Go:** "I will let go of saying yes to social obligations that leave me feeling drained."
- **Action Plan:** Practice polite ways to decline invitations and prioritize downtime for myself.
- **Say No To:** "I will say no to working through lunch breaks."
- **Action Plan:** Schedule a daily lunch break and use it for relaxing activities like a walk or reading.

By following these steps, you can thoughtfully determine what to let go of or say no to in order to enhance your sleep, nutrition, self-care, and movement ultimately boosting your health and vitality.

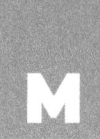 # Saying "No": Your Turn

Now it's your turn… What are you willing to let go or say no to?

28 Days To Declutter Your Home Checklist

When deciding whether to keep an item, ask yourself:
- Have I used this in the past year?
- Does this item bring me joy or serve a purpose?
- Would I buy this again if I didn't already own it?

If the answer to these questions is no, it might be time to let the item go.

- ☐ **Day 1** **Entryway**: Sort through shoes, coats, and accessories. Donate or discard items not worn in the last year.
- ☐ **Day 2** **Entryway**: Organize and clean the entryway closet and storage areas. Add hooks or bins for better organization.
- ☐ **Day 3** **Living Room**: Declutter surfaces like coffee tables, side tables, and entertainment centers. Remove unnecessary decor.
- ☐ **Day 4** **Living Room**: Sort through books, magazines, and DVDs. Donate or recycle items you no longer need.
- ☐ **Day 5** **Living Room**: Organize electronic devices and accessories. Label cords and remove old or unused electronics.
- ☐ **Day 6** **Kitchen**: Go through pantry items, discard expired goods, and donate items you won't use. Organize remaining items by category.
- ☐ **Day 7** **Kitchen**: Declutter kitchen cabinets and drawers. Remove duplicate utensils and appliances. Organize pots, pans, and Tupperware.
- ☐ **Day 8** **Bedroom**: Sort through clothing in closets and drawers. Donate or sell items you haven't worn in the past year.
- ☐ **Day 9** **Bedroom**: Organize accessories, shoes, and bags. Discard damaged items.
- ☐ **Day 10** **Bedroom**: Declutter nightstands, dressers, and under the bed. Clear out old magazines, books, and unnecessary decor.
- ☐ **Day 11** **Kids'/Guest Bedroom**: Sort through toys, books, and clothes. Donate or store outgrown items.
- ☐ **Day 12** **Kids'/Guest Bedroom**: Organize study or play areas. Create designated storage spaces for toys, books, and clothes.
- ☐ **Day 13** **Bathroom**: Go through medicine cabinets and drawers. Discard expired medications and beauty products.

- ☐ **Day 14 Bathroom**: Organize toiletries, towels, and cleaning supplies. Use bins and labels to keep items organized.
- ☐ **Day 15 Home Office**: Sort through paperwork and files. Shred unnecessary documents and organize important ones.
- ☐ **Day 16 Home Office**: Declutter desk drawers and office supplies. Donate or discard unused items.
- ☐ **Day 17 Home Office**: Organize digital files and emails. Delete old files and create a system for ongoing digital organization.
- ☐ **Day 18 Laundry Room**: Sort through cleaning supplies and laundry detergents. Discard empty containers and organize remaining supplies.
- ☐ **Day 19 Laundry Room**: Organize laundry baskets, ironing supplies, and any storage areas. Add shelving or bins if necessary.
- ☐ **Day 20 Hallways and Linen Closets**: Declutter linen closets and hallways. Sort through linens, towels, and blankets. Donate or repurpose items you no longer need.
- ☐ **Day 21 Garage**: Sort through tools, sporting equipment, and seasonal items. Donate or discard unused items.
- ☐ **Day 22 Garage**: Organize storage bins and shelves. Label containers for easy identification.
- ☐ **Day 23 Garage**: Clean and sweep the garage. Create zones for different types of items (e.g., tools, gardening supplies).
- ☐ **Day 24 Basement**: Sort through stored items such as holiday decorations, old toys, and memorabilia. Donate or discard unused items.
- ☐ **Day 25 Basement**: Organize remaining items in labeled bins. Create an inventory list to keep track of what's stored.
- ☐ **Day 26 Attic**: Sort through stored items, similar to the basement. Discard or donate unused items.
- ☐ **Day 27 Attic**: Organize remaining items in labeled bins. Ensure items are properly protected from dust and pests.
- ☐ **Day 28 Final Touches**: Review each room and ensure everything has a designated place. Make final adjustments and enjoy your decluttered home.

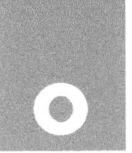

Yellow Light Moment To Self-Care Is A Necessity

How can I optimize my self-care?

_____
_____
_____
_____
_____

What golden nuggets did I take away from this chapter?

_____
_____
_____
_____
_____

What can I start to implement immediately to improve the quality and quantity of my self-care?

_____
_____
_____
_____

Write **3 action steps** and start to implement at least 1 of them this week.

1. _____
   _____
   _____

2. _____
   _____
   _____

3. _____
   _____
   _____

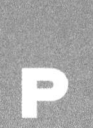 # Movement Questionnaire

Answer the following questions to find out what type of movement you are most likely to stay consistent with.

What challenges me?

_____
_____
_____
_____
_____

What makes me feel confident and strong?

_____
_____
_____
_____
_____

What type of exercise am I most consistent with?

_____
_____
_____
_____
_____

What do I enjoy doing?

_____
_____
_____
_____
_____

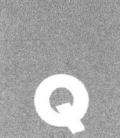

Record Your Waist-To-Hip Ratio

$$\text{WHR} = \frac{\text{Circumfrence Of Waist (inches)}}{\text{Circumfrence Of Hips (inches)}}$$

DATE	WAIST (IN.)	HIPS (IN.)	WHR

Record Your 30 Second Sit-To-Stand Test

Start by sitting in the middle of a chair that does not have arms. The height of the chair should be seventeen inches. Keep your back straight with your feet flat on the floor, approximately shoulder width apart. Now cross your arms at the wrists and hold them against your chest and stand up to a full standing position as many times as you can within a thirty second period. Your score is the total number of stands in that time limit.

DATE	SCORE	DATE	SCORE

FIGURE 6-3: 30 Second Sit-to-Stand Test

AGE	WOMEN	MEN
60–64	< 12	< 14
65–69	< 11	< 12
70–74	< 10	< 12
75–79	< 10	< 11
80–84	< 9	< 10
85–89	< 8	< 8
90–94	< 4	< 7

Yellow Light Moment To Movement Is Key

How can I optimize my movement?

_____
_____
_____
_____
_____

What golden nuggets did I take away from this chapter?

_____
_____
_____
_____
_____

What can I start to implement immediately to improve the quality and quantity of my movement?

_____
_____
_____
_____

Write **3 action steps** and start to implement at least 1 of them this week.

1. _____
_____

2. _____
_____

3. _____
_____

Set Your Goals

Make them Specific, Measurable, Attainable, Relevant, Time-Bound.

S _____

M _____

A _____

R _____

T _____

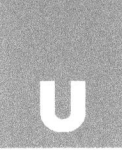# Mind Map Your Challenges

Planning is not about perfection. Planning is the road map needed to guide your steps. Take fifteen minutes to make a plan that would have the most positive impact on your health and wellness right now.

1. Based off your answers on The Vitality Self-Evaluation and Worksheets C, H, O and S, **identify the areas that you feel most challenged by in your vitality journey**. Where do you feel you fall short in keeping your stability? Take five minutes and write your answers in the box labeled Step 1.

2. **Choose one challenge from Step 1 that you feel has the greatest impact on your health and wellness right now.** This is the area that you feel, if you improved, would greatly enhance your vitality. Write that in the circle labeled Step 2.

3. **Outline every obstacle attached to the challenge you wrote in the circle from Step 2.** List every hurdle, no matter how big or small, on the lines projecting from the circle.

4. **Brainstorm every solution you can think of for every obstacle you have just listed in Step 3.** Be creative and think outside of the box—consider every angle. Even if you think the solution is far-fetched and outside of your means, write it down. Ask others to help you brainstorm if you get stuck for ideas. Research solutions if you believe you have ideas outside of your wheelhouse. Jot these solutions next to every obstacle from Step 3.

5. **Turn your solutions into small manageable tasks.** Now that you have concrete ideas on how to overcome your challenges, let's put them into action. Start by picking 1–3 manageable tasks that you feel the most confident with, to get the ball rolling. You are creating a to-do list. This is also a great time to ask others for help with your list. Perhaps they can help you accomplish a specific task. Finding a "WHO" to help you with the HOWs is a great technique when you know something might be outside your reach. This is also an awesome time-management tool.

6. **Give yourself a deadline to start implementing the changes.** Some of the best laid plans are just actions on paper until you start crossing them off the list. Establish a deadline and add it next to each task on your mind map.

7. **Review and adjust accordingly.** This is a working document. Know that you will continue to modify your tasks, obstacles, solutions, and deadlines as you learn what works and what does not. You can assess the effectiveness and efficiency of your plan over time and adjust as your needs change.

Mind Map Your Challenges: Worksheet

STEP 1

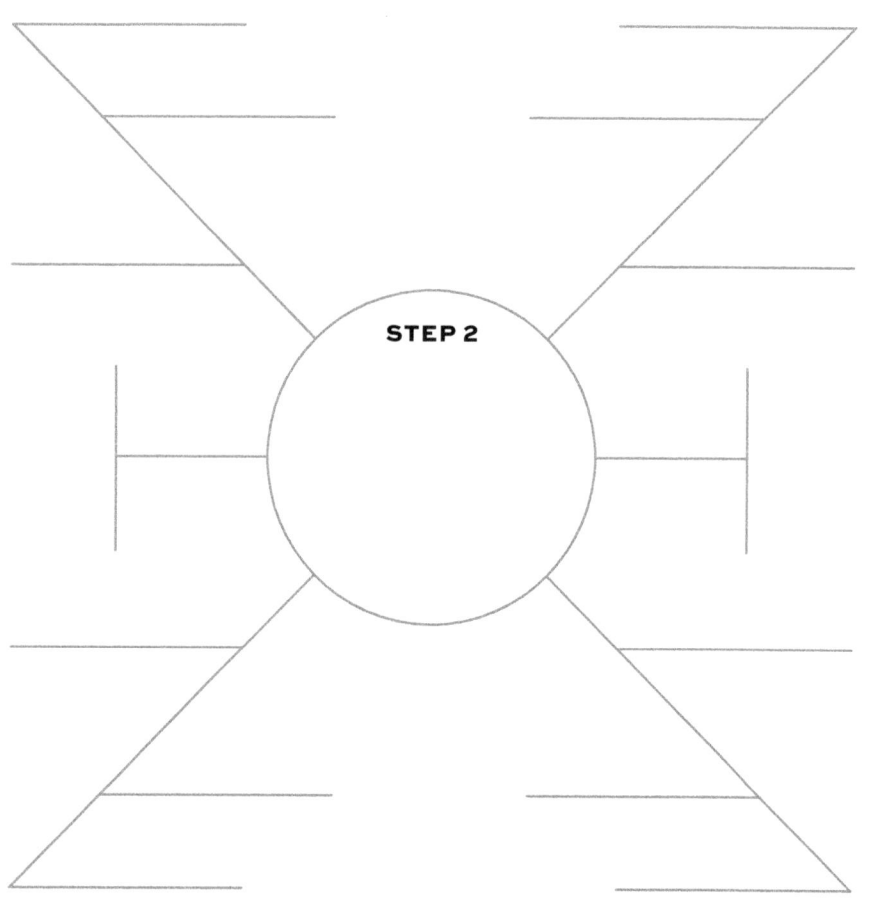

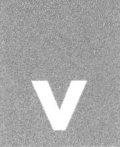

Who You Want To Be

How do you want to be remembered? What legacy do you want to leave behind? This involves introspection and reflection into your values, beliefs, priorities, and joy. Your WHO includes many aspects—personality traits, skills, relationships, and accomplishments in your description. Visualize your WHO. Now write this WHO in the present tense.

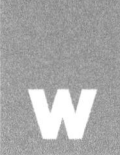

Discover Your Why

Your WHY is the driving force behind everything you do. It is your fundamental motivation. It clarifies your vision, defines your purpose, taps your energy reserves, and sets your motivation into high gear. As you are trying to discover your WHY, consider the following questions:

What golden nuggets did I take away from this chapter?
_____
_____
_____

If time and money were no object, how would you be living your life?
_____
_____

What is your dream job?
_____
_____

What brings you the most joy, makes you feel the most alive, and gets you the most fired up?
_____
_____

What motivates you enough to get up early in the morning and stay up late at night?
_____
_____

What topic can you talk about for hours?
_____
_____

What most excites you during your day?
_____
_____

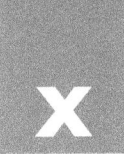

Measure So You Can Manage

Remember: Measuring something is crucial because it provides the necessary data to effectively manage and improve it.

WHAT DO YOU WANT TO MANAGE?	HOW WILL YOU MEASURE YOUR PROGRESS?

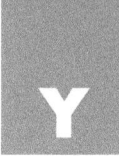 # Control Your Controllables

Understanding and focusing on what you can control in the areas of sleep, nutrition, self-care, and movement can significantly enhance your health and vitality. Here's how to distinguish between what you can and cannot control in these areas:

Steps to Identify Control and Acceptance

1. List Each Area
   - Write down the aspects of sleep, nutrition, self-care, and movement.
2. Divide into Columns
   - Create two columns: "Can Control" and "Can't Control."
3. Brainstorm and Categorize
   - List specific factors under each category for each area. Be honest and specific.
4. Develop an Action Plan
   - For items you can control, write down actionable steps to improve or maintain positive habits.
   - For items you can't control, write down acceptance strategies and alternative plans.
5. Reflect and Adjust
   - Regularly review your lists and action plans. Adjust as needed based on new insights or changes in circumstances.

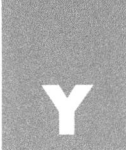# Control Your Controllables: Examples

Sleep

CONTROL
- **Routine:** Set a consistent bedtime and wake-up time.
- **Environment:** Make your bedroom conducive to sleep (quiet, dark, cool, cozy, and calm).
- **Pre-Sleep Habits:** Engage in calming activities before bed (reading, meditation).

CAN'T CONTROL
- **Noise:** Sudden loud noises outside your control (e.g., traffic, neighbors).
- **Stressful Events:** Unexpected events that disrupt your sleep routine.

ACTIONS
- **Control:** Invest in a white noise machine or earplugs to mitigate external noise. Create a wind-down routine to improve sleep quality.
- **Can't Control:** Accept that some nights may be disrupted. Focus on maintaining a consistent routine as much as possible.

Nutrition

CONTROL
- **Food Choices:** Choose whole, nutrient-dense foods.
- **Meal Planning:** Prepare and plan meals in advance.
- **Portion Sizes:** Serve appropriate portion sizes to avoid overeating.

CAN'T CONTROL
- **Availability:** Limited access to certain foods due to location or budget.
- **Social Situations:** Eating out or at events where food choices are limited.

ACTIONS
- **Control:** Create a grocery list of healthy foods, meal prep for the week, and practice mindful eating.
- **Can't Control:** Make the best choices available in social settings and plan for these occasions by eating a healthy snack beforehand.

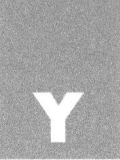

Self-Care

CONTROL
- **Daily Practices:** Set aside time for relaxation and hobbies.
- **Stress Management:** Incorporate stress-relief techniques like deep breathing, meditation, or journaling.
- **Boundaries:** Learn to say no to commitments that overwhelm you.

CAN'T CONTROL
- **External Stressors:** Unexpected events or demands from work or family.
- **Others' Reactions:** How others respond to your boundaries and self-care practices.

ACTIONS
- **Control:** Schedule regular self-care activities and practice mindfulness. Set clear boundaries to protect your time and energy.
- **Can't Control:** Accept that external stressors will occur and focus on how you respond to them. Practice self-compassion and flexibility.

Movement

CONTROL
- **Exercise Routine:** Establish a consistent workout schedule.
- **Types of Activities:** Choose physical activities you enjoy.
- **Daily Activity:** Incorporate movement into your daily routine (e.g., taking the stairs, walking).

CAN'T CONTROL
- **Injuries or Illness:** Physical limitations that temporarily prevent exercise.
- **Weather:** Conditions that might disrupt outdoor activities.

ACTIONS
- **Control:** Create a varied exercise plan that includes both indoor and outdoor activities. Adjust your routine as needed to accommodate changes.
- **Can't Control:** Listen to your body and rest when necessary. Have alternative indoor workouts for bad weather days.

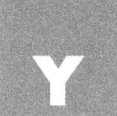

Control Your Controllables: Worksheet

CONTROL	CAN'T CONTROL	ACTION

Do The Dailies

My goal to **thrive** today is: _____
_____

SCULPT IT: Today's Workout

1 hour is only 4% of your day!

Total steps/miles: _____

Ounces of water: _____

FUEL IT: Today's Food

B:

S:

L:

S:

D:

Focus on your fork!

REFLECT ON IT (exercise, nutrition, sleep, stress, water, energy, balance)

The good: _____
The bad: _____
The ugly: _____

PLAN IT & WORK IT (exercise, food plan, sleep/nap, relax/meditate, water)

Tomorrow's goal	Tomorrow's obstacle(s)	Ways to beat obstacle(s)

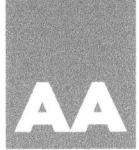 # Prepare Your If... Then Statements

Remember: Having an "if... then" statement is crucial because it establishes clear guidelines for decision-making and actions based on specific conditions or circumstances.

IF...	THEN...

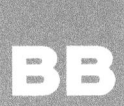

Declare Your Non-Negotiables

Declaring your non-negotiables is important as it sets clear boundaries, ensuring that your values, priorities, and limits are respected in various aspects of your life.

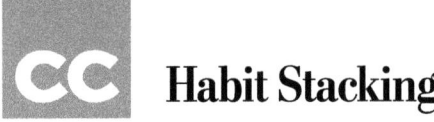

Habit Stacking

EXISTING HABIT	NEW HABIT

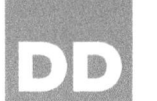 # Habit Tracker

For the next 28 days, I commit to: _____
_____
_____

Check off days as you complete them:

DAY 1	DAY 2	DAY 3	DAY 4	DAY 5	DAY 6	DAY 7
DAY 8	DAY 9	DAY 10	DAY 11	DAY 12	DAY 13	DAY 14
DAY 15	DAY 16	DAY 17	DAY 18	DAY 19	DAY 20	DAY 21
DAY 22	DAY 23	DAY 24	DAY 25	DAY 26	DAY 27	DAY 28

And when I complete all 28 days, my reward is:_____
_____
_____

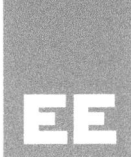

Identify Your Associations and Collaborations

A quick exercise to form associations and collaborations to enhance your health and vitality involves identifying individuals or groups who share similar health goals or interests, reaching out to them via social media, community forums, or local gatherings, and initiating discussions or brainstorming sessions to exchange ideas, provide mutual support, and potentially collaborate on activities such as group workouts, healthy cooking classes, or wellness challenges.

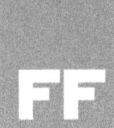

The Vitality Scorecard

Step 1: Evaluate Your Sleep (0-5 Points)
How much sleep and what quality of sleep do you get regularly?

- **5 points:** I sleep 7-9 hours most nights, wake up refreshed, and have a consistent sleep routine.
- **4 points:** I sleep 6-7 hours most nights, have minimal disruptions, and a mostly regular sleep routine.
- **3 points:** I sleep 5-6 hours most nights, but experience occasional interruptions, or have an inconsistent sleep routine.
- **2 points:** I sleep less than 5 hours, it's often poor-quality sleep, or an irregular sleep routine.
- **1 point:** I struggle with falling or staying asleep and often feel exhausted during the day.
- **0 points:** I have severe sleep issues and no regular sleep routine.

SLEEP SCORE: ____ / 5

Step 2: Evaluate Your Nutrition (0-5 Points)
What is the quality of your diet and your eating habits?

- **5 points:** My diet is balanced and nutrient-dense, consisting of a variety of whole foods, and I stay hydrated regularly.
- **4 points:** I mostly eat healthy, with occasional indulgences, and maintain good hydration.
- **3 points:** I sometimes eat processed foods or skip balanced meals and am inconsistently hydrated.
- **2 points:** My diet is unbalanced, often consisting of unhealthy foods, and I don't hydrate enough.
- **1 point:** I rely heavily on processed or fast food, skip meals, and rarely drink water.
- **0 points:** My diet is very unhealthy, with almost no attention to nutrition or hydration.

NUTRITION SCORE: ____ / 5

To download a print-ready copy of The Vitality Scorecard, scan QR code or visit:
jenniephillipscoaching.com/vitality-scorecard

Step 3: Evaluate Your Self-Care (0-5 Points)

Do you spend time on activities that restore your mental and emotional wellbeing?

- **5 points:** I practice self-care like mindfulness, stress relief, and hobbies that make me feel good.
- **4 points:** I practice self-care consistently, but not daily, and focus on my mental well-being most of the time.
- **3 points:** I practice self-care occasionally and try to manage stress or emotional balance.
- **2 points:** I rarely practice self-care and often feel stressed or emotionally drained.
- **1 point:** I rarely practice self-care and frequently feel overwhelmed or burnt out.
- **0 points:** I don't practice self-care and experience significant emotional stress.

SELF-CARE SCORE: _____ / 5

Step 4: Evaluate Your Movement (0-5 Points)

Does your daily activity include structured exercise and strength training?

- **5 points:** I exercise at least 150 min. (moderate intensity) or 75 min. (vigorous intensity) per week with strength training 2-3 times a week.
- **4 points:** I exercise 90-120 min. (moderate intensity) or 45-60 min. (vigorous intensity) per week with strength training 1-2 days a week.
- **3 points:** I exercise 30-60 min. (moderate intensity) or 15-30 min. (vigorous instantly) per week but do not strength train consistently.
- **2 points:** I occasionally exercise, but I have a mostly sedentary lifestyle.
- **1 point:** I am rarely active and live a largely sedentary lifestyle.
- **0 points:** I do not exercise.

MOVEMENT SCORE: _____ / 5

Step 5: Calculate Your Vitality Score

SLEEP	NUTRITION	SELF-CARE	MOVEMENT	VITALITY
☐ +	☐ +	☐ +	☐ =	☐ / 20

Three-Month Refresher

Reassessing your progress three months after setting goals allows you to evaluate your achievements, identify areas of improvement, and adjust your strategies or priorities accordingly. It provides an opportunity for reflection, adaptation, and maintaining momentum towards your long-term objectives, ensuring that you stay focused and accountable on your journey to success.

What are three lessons you have learned so far?

Have you made any shifts (habits, routine, lifestyle) of which you are proud?

What has felt hard or out of sync?

What has been your biggest energy drain?

What habits are no longer serving you?

How will you move forward over the next three months?